Mental Health for Paramedic Science

Mental Health for Paramedic Science

Jo Augustus, Yuet Wah Patrick and Paula Gardner

Open University Press

Open University Press
McGraw Hill
8th Floor, 338 Euston Road
London
England
NW1 3BH

email: enquiries@openup.co.uk
world wide web: www.openup.co.uk

First edition published 2022

A catalogue record of this book is available from the British Library

ISBN-13: 9780335249930
ISBN-10: 0335249930
eISBN: 9780335249947

Library of Congress Cataloging-in-Publication Data
CIP data applied for

Typeset by Transforma Pvt. Ltd., Chennai, India

Praise page

"This is an excellent resource for educators and clinicians around the often difficult and complex subject of mental health in paramedic practice. The chapters are well considered, and the book contains essential information for those working in the paramedic practice field. The book does an excellent job of simplifying and explaining some difficult concepts making it accessible and useful for all. A must read for all paramedics and pre-hospital clinicians."

Gemma Howlett, Principal Lecturer in Paramedic Apprenticeships,
University of Cumbria, UK

"A unique and valuable book to enable paramedics to undertake the daily challenges of providing care and support for patients and service users experiencing mental health difficulties. This book provides contemporary information, and emphasises the key fundamentals of a person centred approach whilst utilising the biopsychosocial model. Mental health assessment can be a daunting prospect, this book highlights key aspects to support assessment and is a timely, diligently presented text."

Clare Keenan, Lecturer in Paramedic Science BSc (Hons),
University of Plymouth, UK

"This is an essential book, written by credible and knowledgeable authors. This text will prove invaluable reading for any paramedic or student paramedic as the topics covered are acutely relevant to the evolving work within paramedicine. The interesting and informative chapters are supported by helpful and practical case studies, which can be used by the reader to further one's understanding. Without doubt, I will be recommending this as a core reading text within the Paramedic Science university module I lead on."

Chris Matthews, Senior Lecturer in Paramedic Science –
University of Brighton, UK and Critical Care Paramedic
Team Leader – South East Coast Ambulance Service

"The awareness that over the course of our lives we all experience mental health and ill-health as well as physical health and ill-health has grown steadily during the last few years. Alongside this growing appreciation has come the awareness that for paramedics especially, the need to develop our understanding of mental health issues is vital - not merely in order to benefit our patients but for our own wellbeing too. An Introduction to Mental Health for Paramedic Science by Jo Augustus, Yuet Wah Patrick and Paula Gardner brings together

a wealth of information and guidance for paramedics and students that I believe will prove to be a valuable resource for understanding and developing care – for both patients and paramedics alike."
Chris Storey, Paramedic and Senior lecturer, University of Brighton

"Have you heard the expression: 'You don't know what you don't know'? As frontline emergency ambulance staff, we encounter and navigate complex mental health presentations on a daily basis – often we fumble our way through based on experience and gut instinct, but wouldn't it be nice to know more? Well, this resource offers exactly that: an effective and applied understanding of mental health and evidence-based practice in the context of paramedic practice. The three experienced authors share their in-depth knowledge, provide practical evidence-based guidance and talk-through applied examples to help us navigate the complex world of mental health – a must have resource for newly qualified and experienced paramedics alike!"
Caitlin Wilson, Paramedic, North West Ambulance Service NHS Trust.
Postgraduate Researcher, University of Leeds, UK

Acknowledgements

Jo Augustus

With thanks to my husband Martin, mum and dad, my inspiration.

Yuet Wah Patrick

To my mum whose upbringing was surrounded by a family plagued with mental health disorders, but nobody ever knew what it was – let's make that change for the future.

Paula Gardner

I would like to thank my partner Richard for inspiring me, and my children Jacob, Cameron, Joseph and Ella who have patiently allowed me the time and space to write. A special thank you to my mum, Rachel, for being a constant support in everything I do.

To my co-authors Jo and Yetti, this has been an amazing journey and I thank you both for making it an enjoyable and memorable experience.

Contents

About the authors

Joanne Augustus

Joanne is a senior lecturer at the University of Worcester in the UK, in the School of Allied Health and Community. She works as Course Leader on the Foundation Degree in Mental Health, and joined the university after ten years working in the NHS and the independent sector in the UK. She provides individual and group-based psychological interventions and has special interests in the treatment of post-traumatic stress disorder, mood disorders, generalized anxiety disorder, low self-esteem, obsessive compulsive disorder, binge eating disorder and bulimia. Post-qualification she has completed training courses in third wave therapies, including eye movement desensitization and reprocessing (EMDR), acceptance and commitment therapy (ACT) and mindfulness.

Paula Gardner

Paula is a senior lecturer at the University of Worcester in the UK, in the School of Allied and Health and Community. She is the Course Leader for the BSc (Hons) Paramedic Science programme, joining the university after 20 years in the ambulance service, and has been an HCPC-registered paramedic since 2001. Her special interests are mental health assessment, resilience, the links between stress and distress, and suicide risk assessment. She has completed postgraduate courses on suicide prevention and supporting and managing those at risk of suicide.

Yuet Wah Patrick

Yuet Wah is a senior lecturer at the University of Gloucestershire, UK. She teaches undergraduate paramedic science with a focus on ethics and law in paramedicine and vulnerable and minority groups. Yuet Wah has been an HCPC-registered paramedic since 2009, and prior to working in higher education she worked for a UK ambulance trust as a paramedic and a clinical team mentor.

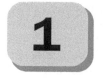

1 Introduction to paramedic science and mental health

Jo Augustus

Depression is lost in the chains that bind
Their release found in stillness of being

Jo Augustus

Introduction

This chapter will explore the aims and structure of the book as well as introducing some of the key concepts and theories.

Aims of the book

As a profession, paramedic science is an essential part of medicine and has seen a diversification of careers within Primary Care. Paramedics are increasingly encountering complex mental health difficulties in practice and in these situations need to provide the most appropriate care pathway. In order to do this, paramedics require an effective understanding of mental health and evidence-based practice in the context of emergency medicine. At the time of writing there are very few key textbooks that adopt such an applied approach to paramedic science. This book is written by three experienced senior lecturers, two of whom have over 20 years' experience each working as paramedics and one of whom is a mental health professional with over 17 years' experience working in primary and secondary care mental health services.

Structure of the book

This book will be underpinned by the principles of person-centred care using the bio-psycho-social model, while emphasizing the importance of taking a whole person approach. Key concepts will be presented in a clear, concise and accessible way. Tables, case studies, diagrams and case discussions will be used to enhance key learning. Legislation principles and practices will be considered in the wider context of multidisciplinary working, including roles and responsibilities. The key characteristics of mental health will be presented, linked to how these can be integrated into the assessment processes as part of everyday practices in paramedic science. The book will explore how complex mental health needs can be addressed through the bio-psycho-social model, as well as the barriers that will be encountered. An understanding of evidence-based practice is an essential part of the paramedic role, and the provision of person-centred care and a working knowledge of referral pathways will be considered. Evidence-based biomedical interventions in mental health will be explored, including side effects and contraindicators. The final chapter will explore trauma-informed care and the impact of this on the workforce, including the concept of resilience. Research will be presented to support each chapter in evidence relevant to paramedic science.

The following outlines each chapter.

Chapter 2 will explore the key legislation to support decision-making required in the individual's best interest. This will include the Mental Health Act, Mental Capacity Act and Human Rights Acts. Ethics considerations will also be introduced to highlight the best interest decision for the individual.

Chapter 3 will explore how mental health difficulties can develop from a bio-psycho-social perspective, including adverse childhood experiences.

Chapter 4 will outline the key characteristics of both common and severe and enduring mental health difficulties.

Chapter 5 will explore the different types of assessment that paramedics use in practice, specific to pre-hospital care.

Chapter 6 is divided into two sections. The first outlines pharmacological interventions, including different types and contraindicators. The second introduces referral pathways into mental health services in both primary and secondary care contexts.

Chapter 7 will explore different styles of communication skills required for resolution of conflict and negotiating with individuals experiencing crisis.

Chapter 8 will focus on breaking bad news and its implications for the individual, family and carer.

Chapter 9 will set out different approaches to trauma in the context of organizations and for individuals.

Bio-psycho-social model

This section outlines the principles of the bio-psycho-social model applied across the life course.

The bio-psycho-social model saw a move away from the traditionalist medical model in the mid-1970s as it was argued that this limited evidence-based

Figure 1.1 Interconnection between the bio-psycho-social components

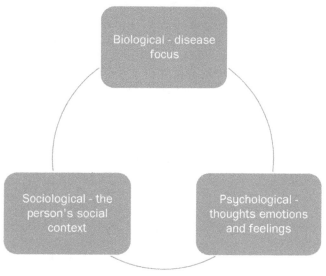

Adapted from Keady et al. 2013

clinical decision-making (Engel 1977). Instead there was a move towards considering health through the lens of the biological, psychological and sociological, as interconnected systems to understand psychiatry (see Figure 1).

In the context of psychiatry this model represents a disruptive interplay between each component of the bio-psycho-social model (Engel 1977). Therefore, from the point of assessment through to recovery the model enables a multidisciplinary and a whole person approach (Engel 1980). The bio-psycho-social model remains established in contemporary mental health practices and is applied to wider disciplines within medicine across the life course (Ghaemi 2010; Keady et al. 2013). As such it has transformed into a philosophy of care and become embedded into the narrative of clinical practice as part of person-centred care approaches (Fava and Sonino 2008; Keady et al. 2013). Therefore the assessment and treatment of mental health should be approached from the perspective of the individual and their situation. However, despite its apparent popularity, the bio-psycho-social model is highly criticized. These criticisms include, but are not limited to, a lack of sensitivity to an individual patient's experience, and a structure that may permit either dominance or subjugation of any of the three components (McLaren 1998; Ghaemi 2010; Benning 2015).

Children and mental health: bio-psycho-social model

Children experiencing medical events often develop symptoms of post-traumatic stress disorder (Balluffi et al. 2004; Kean et al. 2006; Mintzer et al. 2005; Walker et al. 1999). Marsac et al. (2014) proposed a model of bio-psycho-social processes in the peri-trauma period as a way to identify children at risk of developing post-traumatic stress disorder symptoms. The early identification of such symptoms can support the delivery of preventative interventions. A sudden medical event or acute medical events are recognized as those most likely to cause trauma experiences in childhood (Murray and Lopez 1996). The peri-trauma period is typically characterized by physical pain, and contact with medical professionals, including paramedics and treatment. The interactions of all these components can significantly influence the child's internalization of their experiences. The peri-trauma period provides an opportunity to assess and implement preventative interventions (Marsac et al. 2014).

Adult mental health: the bio-psycho-social model

Despite significant advances in the area of mental health there remain some diagnoses that lack understanding in the context of condition development (Strober and Johnson 2012). Anorexia nervosa is one such example, where there is no one effective model of treatment and there is often a recognition of this diagnosis being treatment resistant. Munro et al. (2017) propose a model that adopts an integrative approach as a way to understand the illness as a whole. This provides an opportunity to develop new theoretical approaches that understand the causes, development and continuation of anorexia nervosa to assist professionals in providing effective care pathways. Munro et al.'s (2017) proposed integrative model offers an understanding of the neurobiological, physiological and psychological mechanisms involved in the maintenance of anorexia nervosa, as well as self-critical and shameful experiences associated with the diagnosis. It is therefore hoped that providing clinicians with training in this approach will help reduce hospital admissions.

Dementia care: the bio-psycho-social model

The bio-psycho-social model is an established approach in dementia care, supporting the delivery of evidence-based decision-making (NICE 2018). Such a model of dementia provides a whole person approach that is culturally relevant to the experience of living with dementia and care provision applicable to different settings. The interconnection of the components of the bio-psycho-social model and the dementia journey arguably forms the foundations of effective evidence-based care (Keady et al. 2013). This could include:

- The biological component of the model – the understanding of a change in neurotransmitters and the subsequent impact this has on an individual's cognitive functioning.
- The psychological component of the model – the individual's behaviour as holding meaning relevant to their experience.
- The social model component of the model – the social identity of the individual intrinsic to their sense of self, including self-worth and value. (Adapted from: Sabat (2008).)

Person-centred care

Person-centred care is an established approach that encompasses the capabilities linked to the concept of persons (Entwistle and Watt 2013) – the characteristics of persons, including their physical properties and consciousness, for example. Person-centred care is recognized as using the values and preferences of the individual to guide specific healthcare needs. It is closely aligned to other schools of thought such as humanistic values, and the ability to actively listen (Rogers 1989). Person-centred care focuses on the care needs of the individual, ensuring their preferences, values and needs support the decision-making processes. In addition, the provision of care is respectful and responsive to them (Sundler et al. 2019).

When applied to a specific area of practice such as dementia care, person-centred care requires a holistic approach that recognizes the uniqueness of every individual with dementia (Brooke and Stiell 2018). Kitwood (1997) followed this approach in the development of the concept of personhood, which emphasizes the individual's sense of self while delivering care that seeks to enhance the individual's social world (Choonara and Williams 2021). Personhood emphasizes shared decision-making in practice to develop and maintain quality of care provision (NICE 2018).

Paramedic science in context

Paramedics are first contact practitioners who provide evidence-based pre-hospital care including assessment and treatment in the management of complex cases, often requiring critical care. Working autonomously, paramedics also help to manage distress that may arise from the incident, which may make decision-making more complex (Shields and Flin 2013). Therefore, paramedics require a variety of specific technical and non-technical competencies to fulfil their roles effectively both independently and with the involvement of multi-agency working (Bennett et al. 2021). In clinical simulation Yule et al. (2018) reported that the effective application of non-technical competencies improves performance and subsequently patient safety. Non-technical competencies include – but are not limited to – communication skills, decision-making and teamwork (Bennett et al. 2021). The role of the paramedic operates at the intersection of emergency medicine, public health and public safety (O'Meara et al. 2017). Arguably the role also extends to activities associated with public health prevention, such as education. This intersectionality is essential in the delivery of effective mental health care.

Mental health

Mental health is recognized as an essential component of health – comprised of physical, social and mental well-being – rather than the absence of a mental health diagnosis. WHO (2018) recognizes that mental health is 'a state of well-being in which an individual realizes his or her own abilities, can cope with the normal stresses of life, can work productively and is able to make a contribution to his or her community'.

Poor mental health is connected to discrimination, social exclusion, poor working conditions and social determinants of health such as unhealthy lifestyles and poor physical health, for example. There are various social, psychological and biological factors that influence an individual's mental health, such as genetics, violence and socio-economic deprivation (WHO 2018).

Evidence-based medicine

Evidence-based medicine is the use of contemporary best evidence to inform the clinical decision-making (Sackett et al. 1996). This includes published research evidence, clinical judgement and the patient's values and preferences (Carley et al. 2020). Evidence-based practice requires an organizational culture of inquiry to find and implement ever developing research (Kirk and Nilsen 2016). Therefore, evidence-based practice is more than applying research into practice. Arguably the COVID-19 pandemic has required paramedics to provide both a responsive and flexible evidence-based approach (Carley et al. 2020).

Conclusion

This chapter has introduced some of the key concepts and theories that underpin this book. These include the bio-psycho-social model applied across the life course, person-centred care, as well as what the authors mean by paramedic science, mental health and evidence-based medicine.

References

Balluffi, A., Kassam-Adams, N., Kazak, A., Tucker, M., Dominguez, T. and Helfaer, M. (2004) Traumatic stress in parents of children admitted to the paediatric intensive care unit, *Paediatric Critical Care Medicine*, 5(6): 547–53.

Bennett, R., Mehmed, N. and Williams, B. (2021) Non-technical skills in paramedicine: A scoping review, *Nursing and Health Sciences*, 23(1): 40–52.

Benning T.B. (2015) Limitations of the biopsychosocial model in psychiatry, *Advances in Medical Education and Practice*, 6: 347–352. https://doi.org/10.2147/AMEP.S82937

Brooke, J. and Stiell, M. (2018) Paramedics and dementia, *Journal of Dementia Care*, 26(3): 28–9.

Carley, S., Horner, D., Body, R. and Mackway-Jones, K. (2020) Evidence-based medicine and COVID-19: What to believe and when to change, *Emergency Medicine Journal*, 37(9): 572–5.

Choonara, E. and Williams, J. (2021) What factors affect paramedics' involvement of people with dementia in decisions about their care? A qualitative study, *British Paramedic Journal*, 5(4): 1–8.

Engel, G.L. (1977) The need for a new medical model: A challenge for biomedicine, *Science*, 196(4286): 129–36.

Engel, G.L. (1980) The clinical application of the biopsychosocial model, *American Journal of Psychiatry*, 137(5): 535–44.

Entwistle, V. and Watt, I.S. (2013) Treating patients as persons: A capabilities approach to support delivery of person-centered care, *American Journal of Bioethics*, 13(8): 29–39.

Fava, G.A. and Sonino, N. (2008) The biopsychosocial model thirty years later [biography editorial historical article], *Psychotherapy and Psychosomatics*, 77(1): 1–2. doi:10.1159/000110052.

Ghaemi, S.N. (2010) *The Rise and Fall of the Biopsychosocial Model: Reconciling Art and Science in Psychiatry*. New York: JHU Press.

Keady, J., Jones, L., Ward, R. et al. (2013) Introducing the bio-psycho-social-physical model of dementia through a collective case study design, *Journal of Clinical Nursing*, 22(19–20): 2768–77.

Kean, E., Kelsay, K., Wamboldt, F. and Wamboldt, M. (2006) Posttraumatic stress in adolescents with asthma and their parents, *Journal of the American Academy of Child and Adolescent Psychiatry*, 45(1): 78–86.

Kirk, J. W. and Nilsen, P. (2016) Implementing evidence-based practices in an emergency department: Contradictions exposed when prioritising a flow culture, *Journal of Clinical Nursing*, 25(3–4): 555–65.

Kitwood, T. (1997) *Dementia Reconsidered: The Person Comes First*. London: McGraw-Hill Education.

Marsac, M.L., Kassam-Adams, N., Delahanty, D.L., Widaman, K.F. and Barakat, L.P. (2014) Posttraumatic stress following acute medical trauma in children: A proposed model of bio-psycho-social processes during the peri-trauma period, *Clinical Child and Family Psychology Review*, 17(4): 399–411.

McLaren, N.A. (1998) Critical review of the biopsychosocial model, *Australian and New Zealand Journal Psychiatry*, 32(1): 86–92.

Mintzer, L., Stuber, M., Seacord, D., Castaneda, M., Mesrkhani, V. and Glover, D. (2005) Traumatic stress symptoms in adolescent organ transplant recipients, *Paediatrics*, 115(6): 1640–9.

Munro, C., Randell, L. and Lawrie, S.M. (2017) An integrative bio-psycho-social theory of anorexia nervosa, *Clinical Psychology and Psychotherapy*, 24(1): 1–21.

Murray, C. and Lopez, A. (1996) *The Global Burden of Disease: A Comprehensive Assessment of Mortality and Disability from Diseases, Injuries, and Risk Factors in 1990 and Projected to 2020*. Cambridge, MA: Harvard University Press.

National Institute for Health and Care Excellence (NICE) (2018) *Dementia: Assessment, Management and Support for People Living with Dementia and their Carers [NG97]*. Available at: https://www.nice.org.uk/guidance/ng97 (accessed 28 May 2021).

O'Meara, P.F., Furness, S. and Gleeson, R. (2017) Educating paramedics for the future: A holistic approach, *Journal of Health and Human Services Administration*, 40(2): 219–53.

Rogers, C.R. (1989) *On Becoming a Person*. New York: Houghton Mifflin.

Sabat, S.R. (2008) A bio-psycho-social approach to dementia, in M. Downs and B. Bowers (eds) *Excellence in Dementia Care: Research into Practice*. Maidenhead: Open University Press, pp. 70–84.

Sackett, D.L., Rosenberg, W.M., Muir Gray, J.A., Haynes, R.B. and Richardson, W.S. (1996) Evidence based medicine: What it is and what it isn't, *BMJ*, 312(7023): 71–2. doi:10.1136/bmj.312.7023.71.

Shields, A. and Flin, R. (2013) Paramedics' non-technical skills: A literature review, *Emergency Medicine Journal*, 30(5): 350–4.

Strober, M. and Johnson, C. (2012) The need for complex ideas in anorexia nervosa: Why biology, environment, and psyche all matter, why therapists make mistakes, and why clinical benchmarks are needed for managing weight correction, *The International Journal of Eating Disorders*, 45(2): 155–78.

Sundler, A.J., Hjertberg, F., Keri, H. and Holmström, I.K. (2019) Attributes of person-centred communication: A qualitative exploration of communication with older persons in home health care, *International Journal of Older People Nursing*, 15(1): e12284-n/a.

Walker, A., Harris, G., Baker, A., Kelly, D. and Houghton, J. (1999) Posttraumatic stress responses following liver transplantation in older children, *Journal of Child Psychology and Psychiatry*, 40(3): 363–74.

WHO (2018) *Mental Health: Strengthening our Response*. Available at: https://www.who.int/news-room/fact-sheets/detail/mental-health-strengthening-our-response (accessed 26 May 2021).

Yule, S., Gupta, A., Gazarian, D. et al. (2018) Construct and criterion validity testing of the Non-Technical Skills for Surgeons (NOTSS) behaviour assessment tool using videos of simulated operations, *British Journal of Surgery*, 105(6): 719–27.

2 Legislation and paramedic science

Yuet Wah Patrick

Learning objectives

To identify the key aspects of legal frameworks the paramedic must engage with, including:

- Mental Health Act (1983)
- Places of safety
- Mental Health (Care and Treatment) (Scotland) Act (2003)
- Mental Capacity Act (2005) England and Wales
- Adults with Incapacity (Scotland) Act (2000)
- Mental Capacity Act (Northern Ireland) (2016)
- Best interests
- Restraint
- Human Rights Act (1998)

Introduction

Making decisions and acting in a person's best interests is challenging at the best of times for paramedics, but even more so if the person has a mental health condition and lacks decision-making capacity during a crisis. Paramedics must be equipped to make timely decisions in unpredictable environments while sensitively dealing with people experiencing distressing emotional and mental states. The fact that the paramedic will usually be meeting the service user for the first time when called to an incident, coupled with the possibility that the call is out of hours, making it difficult to gain further information about the person, and the limited pathways that are available for mental health referrals in the acute setting, means that the paramedic has limited resources at hand to make decisions on behalf of the individual who lacks capacity.

The aim of this chapter is to provide an understanding of how legal frameworks are designed to protect and safeguard individuals from harm, and how knowledge of these legislations can enable the paramedic to act appropriately, safely and legally while contemplating the values and preferences of the individual.

The Mental Health Act (1983)

The Mental Health Act (MHA) of 1983 is applicable in England and Wales and comprises a number of 'sections' under which people with a serious mental health condition can be detained for assessment and/or treatment, with or without their consent, if their safety or the safety of others is at risk. It also provides safeguards for patients to ensure they are not inappropriately treated under the provisions of the Act. There is no lower age limit for a person to be detained, however if the person is under 18 there is a duty for them to be placed in a ward that is suitable to their needs according to their age.

The Mental Health Act (2007)

The 2007 MHA is an amendment of the MHA (1983). Key changes include:

- How mental disorder is defined – in the 1983 Act, there were four categories of mental disorders – mental illness, mental impairment, psychopathic disorder and severe mental impairment. The 2007 Act abolished and replaced these categories with a single definition of 'any disorder or disability of the mind'.
- Specific roles of professionals were extended. The role of the Approved Mental Health Professional (AMHP) was created, replacing the Approved Social Worker (ASW), and the Responsible Medical Officer (RMO) was replaced by the Responsible Clinician (RC). A wider range of health professionals are now able to work as AMHPs or RCs providing they have undertaken the appropriate training. These roles are discussed in more detail in Table 2.1 below.
- Patients can request to displace their Nearest Relative (NR) if their existing NR is behaving unreasonably or not in their best interests. Also, civil partner has been added to the list alongside spouse.
- Patients can be detained only if appropriate treatment is available at the time. They cannot be detained if they cannot be treated for their condition.
- The introduction of Supervised Community Treatment (SCT) and Community Treatment Orders (CTOs) allows people who have been sectioned to live in the community if they still need treatment but not in the hospital setting.
- An Independent Mental Health Advocate (IMHA) can support certain eligible patients to challenge any decision they are not happy with.

Multidisciplinary team: roles and responsibilities

Before looking at the different legal frameworks in more detail, it is useful to understand the roles of professionals who may be involved in the welfare of the individual who is undergoing a mental health episode. In brief, a process of *application, assessment and conveyance* is undertaken by different roles.

Certain healthcare professionals, such as an Approved Mental Health Professional (AMHP), or the Nearest Relative (see Table 2.1) can apply for a person to be 'sectioned'. Assessment is carried out by specially trained medical doctors as well as the AMHP to determine if it is appropriate for the person to be detained under 'section' or not. The paramedic is then often requested to transfer the patient from their current location to the receiving institution.

Table 2.1   Roles and responsibilities

Profession	Eligibility
Approved Mental Health Professional (AMHP) An AMHP can assess a person with a mental disorder under the MHA (2007) and recommend for them to be sectioned under the MHA or for a CTO to be administered, if appropriate.	**Who can be an AMHP?** The following professionals can be an AMHP if they have undertaken specialist training in the MHA: • social workers • community mental health nurses • occupational therapists • clinical psychologists Note that a medical practitioner cannot be an AMHP even if they hold any of the qualifications listed.
Section 12(2) approved doctor A section 12(2) approved doctor is a registered medical practitioner who has undertaken approved additional training.	**Who can be a section 12(2) doctor?** Consultant psychiatrist GP Forensic medical examiner
Approved clinician (AC) An AC can carry out certain duties under the MHA, and also have the power to make decisions about a detained person's treatment.	**Who can be an Approved Clinician?** Consultant psychiatrist Medical practitioner (doctor) Mental health or learning disability nurse Occupational therapist Psychiatrist Chartered psychologist Social worker

(Continued)

Table 2.1   (Continued)

Profession	Eligibility
Responsible Clinician (RC) A RC is an experienced medical professional with overall responsibility for the care of a person being treated under the MHA. They will be consulted by other professionals. The RC will decide if a person can be discharged or if their detention under the MHA should be extended. They can also place somebody on a CTO.	**Who can be a Responsible Clinician?** All Responsible Clinicians must be an Approved Clinician – see professions above.
Second opinion appointed doctor (SOAD) A SOAD is required to approve certain decisions about the treatment for a person who is detained under the MHA or given a CTO.	**Who can be a SOAD?** A SOAD should be an independent doctor, who is not involved in the treatment of the individual and is not their RC.
Nearest Relative (NR) The NR is given rights and powers if a person is admitted to hospital under a section of the MHA or subject to a CTO. The NR may request that the person is detained in hospital under the MHA or discharged from hospital. They have the right to be given information about the person's care, and to be consulted on any decisions made.	**Who is the Nearest Relative?** The Nearest Relative is defined by law and is prioritized in the following order: 1. Spouse/civil partner 2. Son or daughter 3. Parent 4. Brother/sister 5. Grandparent If there is more than one person at a given level, for example more than one brother or sister, then the eldest takes priority and is selected as the Nearest Relative.
Police The police play a key role in section 135 and 136 of the MHA. They are responsible for gaining access to a person with a mental disorder and removing them to a place of safety. In some localities, the police work with a paramedic and a nurse to assist people experiencing a mental health crisis in a pre-hospital setting	

(Continued)

Profession	Eligibility
Paramedic Often the first person to deal with a mental health crisis is a paramedic. A paramedic can make an initial health assessment and decide if the person needs any further medical intervention. When a person is 'sectioned' in the community, an ambulance is usually called to transfer the person to the destination hospital or place of safety.	

The Mental Health Act (1983) sections

There are several sections included in the MHA (1983), although the majority are beyond the scope of this book. The sections which will be covered are deemed the most relevant to paramedic practice – these include:

Section 2 – Detention for assessment
Section 3 – Detention for treatment
Section 4 – Admission for assessment in cases of emergency
Section 135 – Warrant to search for and remove patients
Section 136 – Removal of mentally disordered persons without a warrant

Table 2.2

Section 2: Detention for assessment	
Who can be detained under section 2? Anyone who is suffering from a mental disorder who needs to be assessed in a hospital to reduce the risk of them harming themselves or to protect others.	
Who can apply for and approve a section 2 detention? An AMHP **or** the NR can make the application. Approval must be gained from a section 12 approved doctor **and** a second doctor – preferably one who knows the person, such as their GP, or a doctor who has previously dealt with the person. If a GP is not available, then an independent section 12 approved doctor will be consulted.	The **medical recommendation*** must be signed by a section 12 approved doctor **and** a second doctor. The document is to stay with the patient during transit from their home to their destination.

(Continued)

Table 2.2   (Continued)

Section 2: Detention for assessment

How long can a person be detained under section 2?
Up to 28 days unless the RC decides that the person needs to be detained for longer. In this case, an application for detention under section 3 would be made.

* A medical recommendation is a legal document once signed and dated by the medical professionals who have examined and assessed the patient. This document must be conveyed with the patient and handed over to the receiving healthcare institution.

Table 2.3

Section 3: Detention for treatment

Who can be detained under section 3?
A person who needs treatment in a hospital as opposed to in the community for their own protection or the protection of others. Appropriate treatment needs to be readily available for the person to be detained.

Who can apply for and approve a section 3 detention?
An AMHP **or** the NR can make the application.
Approval must be gained from a section 12 approved doctor **and** a second doctor – preferably one who knows the person, such as their GP, or a doctor who has previously dealt with the person.
If a GP is not available, then an independent section 12 approved doctor will be consulted.

The **medical recommendation*** must be signed by a section 12 approved doctor a second doctor.
The document is to stay with the patient during transit from their home to their destination.

How long can a person be detained under section 3?
Up to six months – the RC can apply for an extension of an additional six months and then up to a year.

Information box 2.1 Talking therapies in acute psychiatric inpatient units

Psychological therapies are evidence-based interventions offered to individuals with common and severe and enduring mental health difficulties. They are often referred to as 'talking therapies' and include psychological approaches such as cognitive behaviour therapy, systemic therapy, interpersonal therapy, counselling or dialectical behaviour therapy. These are delivered individually or in a group setting by an experienced psychological therapist who works both collaboratively and non-judgementally with individuals to explore the impact of their difficulties (Augustus et al. 2019). Psychological therapies can therefore be offered to individuals detained under the Mental Health Act, during periods of assessment (Section 2) and treatment (Section 3) (Mental Health Act 2007). Depending on the diagnosis and presentation, the National Institute for Health and Care Excellence (NICE) recommends a minimum of 10–16 sessions of psychological therapy (NICE 2009, 2014). However, given the sometimes short duration of inpatient stays, it can be problematic to achieve the minimum number of recommended sessions. Therefore, the evidence base of providing psychological therapies in acute psychiatric inpatient units is often debated (Jacobsen et al. 2018; Wood et al. 2019). Despite this, there are increasing calls for the consistent provision of psychological therapies in inpatient units, which could include brief psychological therapy (Paterson et al. 2018; Wood et al. 2019).

The use of psychological therapies in acute psychiatric inpatient units is often associated with improvements in psychological distress and a reduction in admissions to hospital (Paterson et al. 2018). Individuals being detained under the Mental Health Act should be offered the least restrictive intervention as outlined in the Mental Health Act: Code of Practice (Sustere and Tarpey 2019). For example, Jacobsen et al. (2018) recognize that psychological therapies can be effectively used alongside medication and nursing care. Sustere and Tarpey (2019) identified that psychosocial interventions could include engagement in meaningful activities that are similar to daily life, arguably acting to provide the least restrictive approach – and also reducing the use of isolation and encouraging positive risk-taking behaviours. This could address the failings identified in the delivery of care in acute psychiatric inpatient units (Wood et al. 2019). Such failings were identified in the Government's *Five Year Forward View* (Department of Health and Social Care 2017) and the Mental Health Act review (Department of Health 2018), including the need to deliver interventions that act to prevent hospital admissions (Wood et al. 2019).

Table 2.4

Section 4: Admission for assessment in cases of emergency

Who can be detained under section 4?
A person who needs *urgent* admission to hospital for an assessment of a suspected mental disorder.
An application for detention under section 4 may be made only when:

- the criteria for detention for assessment under section 2 are met **and**
- the patient's detention is required as a matter of urgent necessity **and**
- obtaining a second medical recommendation would cause undesirable delay.

(Continued)

Section 4: Admission for assessment in cases of emergency

To be satisfied that an emergency has arisen, the person making the application and the doctor making the supporting recommendation should have evidence of:

- an immediate and significant risk of mental or physical harm to the patient or to others
- danger of serious harm to property **or**
- a need for the use of restrictive interventions on a patient.

It should be noted that it is rare that a section 4 is applied for, as a section 2 detention should be sought whenever possible.

Who can apply for and approve a section 4 detention?
An AMHP **or** the NR can make the application.
Approval must be gained from a section 12 approved doctor **or** a doctor who knows the person, such as their GP, or who has previously dealt with the person.

The **medical recommendation*** document needs to be signed by **one** doctor.
Only one doctor needs to provide a medical recommendation under section 4 if waiting for a second doctor's signature will cause delay and will be detrimental to the health and welfare of the person to be detained or to others.
Once a second doctor's signature has been obtained then the section 4 detention turns into a section 2 detention.

How long can a person be detained under section 4?
Up to 72 hours.

Table 2.5

Section 135: Warrant to enter and search for a person with a mental disorder

Who can be detained under section 135?
There are two different situations where somebody may be detained under section 135.
A person believed to be suffering from a mental disorder who is in a private place **and**:

1 is being ill-treated or neglected or is unable to care for themselves
   or
2 has left a place where they were detained under the Mental Health Act without permission.

The person can be taken to a place of safety from a private dwelling.

Who can apply for a section 135 detention?
An AMHP can make the application.

An application is made to the Magistrates' Court for a warrant to allow police officers to enter a private premises.

(Continued)

Section 135: Warrant to enter and search for a person with a mental disorder

The AMHP may ask for a warrant if:

- it is likely that healthcare professionals will be denied access to the private dwelling
- there is a risk of violence
- there is a risk the detainee will abscond before the assessment is completed
- the detainee is likely to self-harm

or

- there is a risk that a pet, such as a dog, will attack the AMHP.

The warrant allows the police and healthcare professionals to enter a private property if there is a concern for someone's mental health and welfare, even if it is against the person's wishes.

The person can then be taken to a place of safety as deemed necessary.

Under section 135(1), the police, an AMHP and a doctor (does not have to be s12 approved) must be present.

Under section 135(2), the police can attend alone but they are encouraged to bring someone from the local hospital or social services with them.

How long can a person be detained under section 135?

Up to 36 hours.

It is unlikely for a paramedic to be involved in detaining someone under section 135. However, it is possible that they may be called to somebody who is eligible for detention under this section, and therefore they should notify the appropriate services for assessment.

Table 2.6

Section 136: Removal of mentally disordered persons without a warrant

Who can be detained under section 136?

A mentally disordered person who is in a public place and 'in need of immediate care or control' and needs further assessment by an approved doctor or an AMHP.

Who can enforce a section 136 detention?

A police officer can enforce a section 136.

The police can remove a person from a public place and take them to a place of safety.

The police officer does not need medical evidence to trigger section 136 but they must check with a health professional, if practicable, before they can enforce it.

The health professionals they could speak to are:

- a medical practitioner, such as a doctor
- a nurse

What is classed as a public place?

Any place *other than* a house, flat or room where a person is living, or a garden or garage that only one household has access to.

(Continued)

Table 2.6   (Continued)

- an AMHP
- an occupational therapist

or

- a paramedic

How long can a person be detained under section 136?
Up to 36 hours:
24 hours initially, with an additional 12 hours if an extension is requested.

A place of safety

There is often much debate in the pre-hospital setting as to which locations are acceptable as a place of safety. The MHA (1983) clearly states that the following locations that can be considered as a place of safety:

- Residential accommodation provided by social services
- A hospital
- A police station (but only in very limited circumstances)
- An independent hospital or care home for mentally disordered persons
- 'Any other suitable place', with the agreement of the person who appears to the police officer to be 'responsible for the management of the place' – this can include someone's home, provided the person thought to be suffering from a mental disorder agrees and (if it is not their own home or they live with others) another person living there also agrees.

It has been highlighted that, in practice, health-based places of safety will generally be the best option:

> The expectation remains that, with limited exceptions, the person's needs will most appropriately be met by taking them to a 'health-based' place of safety – a dedicated section 136 suite where they can be looked after by properly trained and qualified mental health and other medical professionals. (DOH 2017)

Police station

People detained under sections 135 or 136 must be kept at a place of safety until a mental health assessment has been completed. In the past, police stations have been used as a place of safety to detain people, including children and young adults (CQC 2014). Being detained in a police cell can be a terrifying experience, and evidence suggests that unfortunately, due to the lack of available alternative places of safety, or providers not accepting people under the influence of drugs and/or alcohol, police stations were commonly and inappropriately used as a place of safety, which has a negative impact on a person's already fragile mental health (CQC 2014).

Recent changes detailed in the MHA (1983) (Places of Safety Regulations (2017) under section 136A (1)) prohibit the use of police stations as a place of safety for anyone under 18 years old, and stipulate that people can only be detained at a police station for the following reasons:

(i) The behaviour of the person poses an imminent risk of serious injury or death to themselves or another person.
(ii) Because of that risk, no other place of safety in the relevant police area can reasonably be expected to detain them.
(iii) So far as reasonably practicable, a healthcare professional will be present at the police station and available to them.

Hospital

A hospital is deemed a suitable place of safety by the MHA (1983). Dedicated s136 suites are often situated in a non-acute hospital setting where the person can be assessed by a health professional in a secure and private environment.

There is frequent discussion among ambulance staff about the suitability of using an emergency department (ED) as a place of safety. It is useful to note here that the difference between taking somebody to an ED as a place of safety under the detention of s135 or s136 and taking somebody who is not under detention of a section, is that the person under section is obliged to stay and be assessed, by law. This means that additional measures are put into place to ensure that the person does not abscond. The police must always accompany the person to an ED and should stay with them until the safety and security of the individual can be ensured (RCEM 2017 and DOH 2015).

Ambulance staff taking somebody suffering a mental health crisis who is not under section to an ED should be aware that the person is permitted to self-discharge as there is no legal requirement for them to stay. If a person is conveyed to an ED for medical attention and they are deemed to lack decision-making capacity, then every effort should be made to reduce the risk of the person absconding, which could include restraint if necessary. If the person who lacks capacity under the MCA does abscond from an ED, then hospital security staff should search for the person. If they cannot be found, the police should be notified and asked to perform a welfare check. The police are not permitted to bring the person back to an ED against the person's wishes unless they are under s136 (RCEM 2017).

What role does the paramedic play?

Although paramedics are not directly involved in the decision-making to detain a person under the MHA (with the exception of s136), they will frequently encounter people being detained, as the paramedic's primary role, in this case, is conveyance. Therefore, an awareness of the different sections of the MHA will enable the paramedic to deliver person-centred care as the MHA stipulates that 'Patients should always be transported in the manner which is most likely to preserve their dignity and privacy consistent with managing any risk to their health and safety or to other people' (DOH 2015).

This applies in all cases where patients are compulsorily transported under the Act, including:

- Taking patients to hospital to be detained for assessment or treatment
- Transferring patients between hospitals
- Returning patients to hospital if they are absent without leave
- Taking community patients or patients who have been conditionally discharged to hospital on recall

The vast majority of conveyances are without incident. However, there are times when the patient may show signs of aggression or violence. In these circumstances it is wise to request police assistance if they are not already present and if possible, to maintain the person's dignity, the person should be conveyed via ambulance with a police officer in the back with the attending ambulance staff.

If it is necessary to convey the person in the police vehicle due to the risk involved, it may be appropriate for the most highly qualified member of the ambulance crew to sit with the patient, with any medical equipment they may need to deal with any emergencies. The ambulance should follow the police vehicle in case assistance is required (DOH 2015).

Mental Health (Care and Treatment) (Scotland) 2003

The 1984 Mental Health (Scotland) Act was replaced by the Mental Health (Care and Treatment) (Scotland) Act 2003 which came into effect in 2005. This has since been amended by the Mental Health (Scotland) Act 2015. The main benefits of the 2003 Act include the right to access independent advocacy, the appointment of a named person who will support and protect the individual, the provision for advance statements and the protection of the Mental Health Tribunal, which makes decisions and reviews care plans and cases.

The provisions of this Act are intended to ensure that care and compulsory measures of detention (detailed under civil compulsory powers) can be used only when there is a significant risk to the safety or welfare of the patient or other people.

The Scottish Parliament wished to explore the ethical basis of compulsory treatment and to set out recommendations for new Scottish mental health legislation. This led to the development of a set of principles, known as the 'Millan Principles', which underpin the 2003 Act and must be adhered to by any healthcare professional implementing the Act. They encourage non-discrimination, respect for diversity and equality, as well as the involvement of the patient and their family and carers.

Civil compulsory powers

Three main types of civil compulsory powers exist which enforce the assessment and treatment of a person with a mental health disorder. They are:

- A compulsory treatment order (CTO)
- A short-term detention certificate (STDC)
- An emergency detention certificate (EDC)

Compulsory treatment order (CTO)

What is a CTO for?

A CTO is used for the treatment of a person with a mental disorder over a long period of time, either in hospital or at home or another community setting.

Who has the authority to grant a CTO?

An application is made by the Mental Health Officer (MHO), which is then considered by the Mental Health Tribunal. The application must be accompanied by:

- two mental health reports
- the MHO's report, and
- a proposed care plan

The Mental Health Tribunal can grant a CTO after a rigorous application process involving the patient, their named person and the multidisciplinary team.

How long does a CTO last for?

Six months from when it was first granted, then for a further six months if extended, after which it may be extended for a further 12 months and thereafter every 12 months.

Short-term detention certificate (STDC)

What is an STDC for?

An STDC is used where a person is not willing to be admitted to hospital, if they may have a mental disorder that is affecting their judgement about treatment and admission is required for further **assessment and/or treatment** over a short period of time.

Who has authority to grant an STDC?

An STDC may only be granted by an approved medical practitioner if the individual meets certain criteria listed in s44(4) of the Act.

How long does an STDC last for and when does it start?

Up to 28 days from the time the individual arrives at hospital.
An extension can be requested if there is a pending application for a CTO.

Emergency detention certificate (EDC)

What is an EDC for?

An EDC is used when a person is not willing to be admitted to hospital but needs immediate admission for **assessment** (not treatment) of a possible mental disorder and there is not enough time, or no approved medical practitioner available, to apply an STDC. The person must present a significant risk to themselves or to others and is likely to be suffering from a mental disorder.

Who can grant an EDC?

Any registered medical practitioner. The medical practitioner who grants the EDC must be the same one who carries out the examination.

How long does an EDC last for and when does it start?

Up to 72 hours once the person is admitted to hospital.

The Mental Health (Scotland) Act 2015

The Mental Health (Scotland) Act 2015 is an amendment of the Mental Health (Care and Treatment) (Scotland) 2003 Act.
The key changes include:

- The removal of the appointment of named persons by default, so that adult patients only have a named person if they choose to have one (this does not apply to patients under 16).
- The removal of the power of the Tribunal to appoint or substitute a named person for adult patients, and named persons are now required to agree in writing to taking on the role.
- The introduction of a requirement for NHS Boards to keep a copy of any advance statement received with the patient's records and to provide certain information about the existence and location of the statement to the Mental Welfare Commission, to be held on a register of information.
- Some changes of detention provisions. For example, for compulsory treatment orders (CTO), the maximum allowed detention will now be 200 days in any 12-month period, excluding any period of less than eight hours.

The Mental Capacity Act (MCA) 2005 – England and Wales

What is the MCA?

The Mental Capacity Act (MCA) (2005) protects adults aged 16 and above, living in England and Wales, who lack the mental capacity to make particular decisions for themselves. In Scotland, the equivalent is the Adults with Incapacity law (2000) and in Northern Ireland it is the Mental Capacity Act (Northern Ireland) (2016).

The MCA (2005) promotes an individual's autonomy, empowering them to make decisions about their care and planning for their future if they should ever lose decision-making capacity at any time. If a person is deemed not to have decision-making capacity at a given time, then the person who is providing their care must comply with the MCA (2005) and base any decisions on the individual's best interests.

It should be assumed that an adult has the capacity to make decisions for themselves unless it can be proven otherwise. It is equally important to support someone to enable them to make their own decisions. This involves taking steps such as making sure the relevant information is presented or communicated to them in a way that they can understand.

So, what does the term 'a person who lacks capacity' mean? The MCA (2005) Code of Practice states that:

> it means a person who lacks capacity to make a particular decision or take a particular action for themselves at the time the decision or action needs to be taken ... people may lack capacity to make some decisions for themselves, but will have capacity to make other decisions. (Department for Constitutional Affairs 2007)

For example, they may have capacity to make small decisions about everyday issues such as what to wear or what to eat but lack the capacity to make more complex decisions about what treatment they would like to receive. It also reflects the fact that a person who lacks capacity to make a decision for themselves at a certain time may be able to make that decision at a later date. This may be the case for somebody who is intoxicated or unconscious, which is often how a person presents in an emergency. It is therefore essential that the paramedic has a sound understanding of the MCA and how it should be applied in the challenging environment in which they operate.

The MCA (2005) is underpinned by five key principles; the first three should be considered before determining if a person lacks capacity, and the last two are to aid decision-making once it has been established that the person does lack capacity. In order to assess if a person does have decision-making capacity, a two-stage assessment process must be followed – this is discussed in Chapter 5.

The five statutory principles are:

1   A person must be assumed to have capacity unless it is established that they lack capacity.
2   A person is not to be treated as unable to make a decision unless all practicable steps to help them to do so have been taken without success.
3   A person is not to be treated as unable to make a decision merely because they make an unwise decision.
4   An act done, or decision made, under this Act for or on behalf of a person who lacks capacity must be done, or made, in their best interests.
5   Before the act is done, or the decision is made, regard must be had to whether the purpose for which it is needed can be as effectively achieved in a way that is less restrictive of the person's rights and freedom of action.

How should the statutory principles be applied?

Principle 1: *Decision-making capacity should always be assumed unless there is a reason to suggest otherwise.*

Assuming a person has decision-making capacity should always be the starting point of any assessment. A person's autonomy should always be at the forefront of any actions undertaken, and the healthcare professional should not purposely look to refute that the person has decision-making capacity purely because they are not compliant with any advice or treatment plans that the healthcare professional may suggest.

Principle 2: *A person should be supported to make their own decisions.*

The aim of this principle is to promote a vulnerable person's autonomy. Steps should be taken to support the person to make their own decisions without being pressurized or coerced.

The healthcare professional may need to find different forms of communication or use visual aids as a tool. Using layman's terms to help the individual make an informed decision is important. The individual may need medical treatment to calm them or ease their discomfort before they can think rationally. For example, a person who is distressed and in pain may not consent to any further treatment until they have been calmed and their pain is managed.

In emergency situations, if treatment cannot be delayed while a person gets support to make a decision, the only practical and appropriate steps might be to keep a person informed of what is happening and why.

Principle 3: *A person has the right to make unwise decisions.*

Today's society is made up of a wealth of diverse individuals whose own experiences and beliefs shape their values, preferences and attitudes. One person's wishes may be difficult for another person to understand or respect. Healthcare professionals may face dilemmas which make them feel uncomfortable when they attend a person who refuses what they deem the best or most appropriate treatment for their situation.

But as long as the person has the capacity to make the decision and they have been given sufficient information to allow them to make an informed decision, then their decisions must be respected, wise or unwise.

However, if somebody:

- repeatedly makes unwise decisions that put them at significant risk of harm or exploitation, or
- makes a particular unwise decision that is obviously irrational or out of character

then, as far as possible, steps should be taken to rule out any underlying reasons that may be the potential cause of this behaviour.

Principle 4: *Best interests.*

A person's best interests must be the basis for all decisions made and actions carried out on their behalf in situations where they lack capacity to make those particular decisions for themselves. It is not always easy to know what the best interests for each individual are – this will be discussed further later on in this chapter.

Principle 5: *The least restrictive alternative should always be sought.*

Any action to be taken should be the least invasive or interfere the least with the person's basic rights and freedom. This could result in no action being taken at all if that is considered safe and appropriate for the individual. Conversely, depending on the circumstances, it may be that the best option is not to adopt the least restrictive alternative if it is in the best interests of the person.

Adults with Incapacity (Scotland) Act 2000

The Adults with Incapacity (Scotland) Act 2000 aims to protect people aged 16 and over who lack capacity to make particular decisions regarding their welfare and finances due to mental illness, learning disability, dementia or a related condition, or an inability to communicate. It supports their involvement in making decisions about how they wish to live their life and what treatment they would like to receive, as far as they are able to do so.

For the purposes of the Act, 'incapacity' means incapable of making, communicating or understanding decisions or retaining information in order to make decisions due to a mental disorder, or inability to communicate due to a physical disability (Adults with Incapacity (Scotland) Act 2000, s1 (6)).

There are five guiding principles the healthcare professional must consider when acting on behalf of an adult lacking decision-making capacity:

- **Principle 1**: *Benefit* – Actions or decisions made must be to benefit the person and only be taken if that particular action is the only way to achieve that benefit.
- **Principle 2**: *Minimum intervention* – Actions or decisions should be the least restrictive for the individual.

- **Principle 3**: *Wishes of the adult must be considered* – present and past wishes and feelings of the person should be weighed in decision-making.
- **Principle 4**: *Consultation with relevant others* – The views of significant others, such as the nearest relative, primary carer, named person, lasting power of attorney, should be sought if reasonable and practicable to do so.
- **Principle 5**: *Encourage the adult to exercise residual capacity* – The person should be encouraged to use their existing skills in any decision-making in so far as it is reasonable and practicable to do so.

Emergencies

In an emergency, treatment is to be given to an incapacitated adult where consent cannot be obtained to save life and to prevent deterioration.

The Mental Capacity Act (Northern Ireland) (2016)

The Mental Capacity Act (Northern Ireland) (2016) replaces the Mental Health (Northern Ireland) Order (1986) and fuses together mental capacity and mental health law for those aged 16 years old and over within a single piece of legislation. It provides a statutory framework for people who lack capacity to make a decision for themselves at a given time, and for those who currently have capacity but wish to make preparations for the future, if they were to ever lack capacity.

Part one of the Act is underpinned by five principles which the healthcare professional is obliged to adhere to. Assessment of mental capacity also falls under this section. Both the principles and assessment of capacity align closely to the principles and assessment outlined in the MCA (2005) for England and Wales, so will not be repeated here.

Part two of the Act allows the legal deprivation of liberty (DoL) to be undertaken for people who lack capacity. It also protects the professionals who are depriving a person of their liberty, including under emergency situations. It states that emergency action, such as deprivation without delay, can be taken without applying additional safeguards, if a delay would risk unnecessary harm to the individual. The additional safeguards include:

A) **Formal assessment of capacity** – If a person is deemed incapacitated through the mental capacity assessment, a formal statement of incapacity must be made if a DoL is to be granted. This statement can be provided by the following health professionals: a social worker; a medical practitioner; a nurse or midwife; an occupational therapist; a practitioner psychologist; a dentist; or a speech and language therapist. A paramedic cannot make a formal assessment of capacity.

B) **Nominated person (NP)** – The NP is consulted when making a best interest decision. The health professional applying for a DoL must consult the NP for them to be protected from liability. The only exception is if a DoL is sought under emergency conditions and seeking NP approval risks harm caused due to the delay. The NP can be appointed by the individual to be detained if they have the capacity to do so. It is important to note that the person may lack capacity for a DoL decision but may have capacity to appoint an NP. If an NP is not appointed then the NP default list is to be observed. The order of the list is similar to the NR (see Table 2.1), with the exception of 'carer' being at the top of the NP list for Northern Ireland.

C) **Prevention of Serious Harm (POSH) condition** – If the health professional believes that failure to detain a person would create a serious risk of harm to themselves or to others then they can apply for a DoL. The likelihood of harm and its seriousness must be proportionate to the detention.

D) **Authorization** – Authorization for a DoL can be sought in two ways: trust panel authorization and short-term detention.

Trust panel authorization can detain a person in a setting where they can be treated, such as a health or social care setting or in their own home. This also applies to emergency detention. The trust panel must make a decision within seven days of the application to refuse or grant the request. The criteria for authorization of a DoL are as follows:

a. lack of capacity;
b. best interests;
c. appropriate care or treatment is available in the place; and
d. prevention of serious harm condition. (DOH 2019)

Detention under a trust panel authorization can last for a maximum of six months and then may be extended for a further six months, and then for one year. The detained individual can be taken to the receiving unit by anyone, including police officers.

A short-term detention can only be applied in a hospital setting for examination or examination followed by treatment. If the person is in an out-of-hospital setting and needs to be detained during an emergency situation, they can be held for as long as it takes to obtain a trust panel authorization, providing the criteria for a DoL under emergency is met at all times.

Short-term detention authorization can last for a maximum of 28 days.

Case study 2.1

You attend Kelly, a 28 year old homeless female, who is sleeping on the streets. A passer-by has called for an ambulance as she noticed that Kelly was bleeding heavily from her arm. Kelly admits that she has self-harmed, and on examination you see that she has a deep laceration to her left arm. You dress the wound and it stops bleeding, but you are concerned that it is unstable and could easily start to bleed again at any time.

Kelly is calm and chats to you freely as you treat her wound. There is no evidence to lead you to suspect that she has been drinking or taking drugs. You advise her that she will need to attend hospital for stitches. She refuses to go because she does not like the way she is made to feel at hospitals.

Referring to the five principles of the MCA, explain any decisions you may make regarding Kelly's care.

Principle 1 states that a person must be assumed to have capacity unless it is established that they lack capacity. This is the starting point of the MCA (2005). There are no grounds for taking Kelly to ED by force as there is no reason to believe she lacks capacity due to her mental state or from her actions.

Principle 2 says that the person should be supported to help them make their own decisions. In this case, Kelly should be informed of the implications of her actions (blood loss) and the consequences of her decision not to receive further treatment at hospital (further blood loss, infection or unconsciousness). It is important that when Kelly is given this information she is not intimidated or coerced into making a decision.

Principle 3 states that a person is allowed to make unwise decisions. Because a person self-harms does not necessarily mean that they lack capacity. It is possible that Kelly lacked capacity momentarily when she cut herself in the heat of the moment, but she may now have regained capacity as she has had time to collect her thoughts. The actions of the paramedic can only be based on the capacity that the person possesses at the time of the assessment. Kelly does not give reason to suspect that she lacks capacity at the time the paramedic sees her; the paramedic cannot act retrospectively (because she may have lost capacity in the past) or prospectively (she may lose capacity in the future) and take her to ED.

If it was thought that Kelly did lack capacity to refuse treatment, then she could be forced to go to hospital against her wishes. In this case, principles 4 and 5 need to be considered.

Principle 4 advises that any decisions should be made in the person's best interests. Kelly needs to have stitches to stop the wound bleeding again. Her living circumstances mean it will be difficult for her to keep the wound clean, thus increasing the risk of infection. However, her negative previous experience of attending hospital needs to be considered, as any additional similar experiences could potentially further impact on her mental health.

Principle 5 declares that the least restrictive alternative must be taken. In Kelly's case, as she will have to be taken to hospital against her will, this must be conducted in a dignified manner. The paramedic will need to draw on their professional and interpersonal skills to encourage Kelly to accompany them to hospital. If it is thought that Kelly is suffering from a *mental disorder*, the police can be called to assist and potentially enforce section 136 as Kelly is in a public place and is a risk to herself. Consideration should be given to the fact that any police presence may escalate the situation, and they should be asked to attend only as a last resort. If Kelly is *not* thought to be suffering from a mental disorder then section 136 *cannot* be enforced.

Best interests

One of the key principles of the MCA (2005) is to make decisions in a person's best interests. But the fast-paced and unpredictable nature of the pre-hospital setting can make understanding a person's best interests a challenging feat.

Certain principles must be considered when acting in someone's best interests (CQC 2011), as detailed below:

Avoid discrimination – someone's age, appearance, condition or behaviour should not influence judgement.

Every effort should be made to encourage and enable the person to take part in making the decision – this involves communicating in a way that the person understands, if necessary using visual aids, an interpreter or sign language, for example.

Consider all relevant circumstances personal to the individual – how does the proposed treatment impact on the individual's well-being in this particular circumstance? For example, if they are advised to go to hospital for further assessment but they refuse – what are the consequences if they don't go?

Will the person regain decision-making capacity? – if there is a chance that they will, then it may be possible to put off the decision until later if it is not urgent. In emergency situations, it may not be possible to wait to see if the person may regain capacity. It depends on the circumstances and the urgency of treatment. For example, someone who is intoxicated and refuses to have stitches to a laceration on their hand can wait until they are sober to decide on their treatment. However, if the bleeding is limb- or life-threatening then clearly it is not in their best interests to wait for them to sober up to gain their consent, and the paramedic will act accordingly, even if it is against the person's wishes.

The person's past and present wishes and feelings, beliefs and values should be taken into account – ADRT, ReSPECT forms, advance statements, care plans and verbal wishes are documents that can greatly help the paramedic know what the person's wishes are and aid them to act in their best interests.

The views of other people who are close to the person who lacks capacity should be considered, including anyone caring for the person, close relatives and friends, and any attorneys appointed under a lasting power of attorney or enduring power of attorney and/or deputies appointed by the Court of Protection to act for the person.

Special considerations apply to decisions about life-sustaining treatment – the fundamental rule is that anyone who is deciding whether or not life-sustaining treatment is in the best interests of someone who lacks capacity to consent to or refuse such treatment must not be motivated by a desire to bring about the person's death, even if this is from a sense of compassion. All reasonable steps which are in the person's best interests should be taken to prolong their life. There will be a limited number of cases where treatment is futile, overly burdensome to the patient, or where there is no prospect of recovery. In circumstances such as these, it may be that an assessment of best interests leads to the conclusion to withdraw or withhold life-sustaining treatment, even if this may result in the person's death.

Restraint

What is restraint?

Section 6(4) of the MCA (2005) states that someone is using restraint if they:

* use force – or threaten to use force – to make someone do something they are resisting, or
* restrict a person's freedom of movement, whether they are resisting or not

Restrictive practice or restraint has been explained as 'making someone do something they don't want to do or stopping someone doing something they want to do' (Skills for Care and Skills for Health 2014).

Restraint comes in various forms, including:

Verbal – coercion or verbal intimidation is used to persuade someone to do something or to stop someone from carrying out an action
Physical – physical contact is used: this could be physically blocking an exit or grabbing someone to stop them from hitting another person
Mechanical – equipment such blankets and straps are used to prevent movement
Chemical – medication is used to sedate the person – not in paramedic scope
Environmental – isolation, such as locking someone in a room or the back of the ambulance to keep them contained

Paramedics use restraint on a regular basis, often unwittingly. Wrapping someone in a blanket and strapping them into a carry chair or holding someone's arm while cannulating are examples of restraint.

Restraint is a practice that should be used as a last resort but it is useful to know the legal and ethical implications it may involve when used.

When is it necessary to use restraint?

A person may be lawfully restrained under the MCA (2005) if the following criteria are met:

* The person lacks capacity and restraint is in their best interests
* It is necessary to prevent harm to the person
* The amount or type of restraint used and the amount of time it lasts must be a proportionate response to the likelihood and seriousness of harm

A paramedic may have to restrain a person if they are resisting being taken to a place of safety such as a hospital, for example, or to prevent them from absconding en route; or they may be refusing vital medical treatment. A person may also be restrained under common law if they pose a risk to themselves or to others. The Department for Constitutional Affairs (2007) states that restraint should never be used if the sole aim is to make it easier to perform a particular task.

What steps should be taken to restrain a person?

The least restrictive method should always be employed and for the minimum amount of time. In most cases, restraint can be avoided by verbal de-escalation, and prevention is always the preferred method. Nevertheless, there are times when verbal de-escalation is either ineffective or, in the case of a dangerous or aggressive person, inappropriate. In this case, the next least restrictive method should be considered, which may be physical or mechanical restraint.

Restraint must always be proportionate to the risk posed and only reasonable force should be used. As there is no legal definition of 'reasonable force', it does allow for interpretation, but it is essential that any restraint used must be documented and justified. If a restraint method appears inappropriate to the threat posed, then the person is being unlawfully restrained. For example, if a person is having a seizure and the paramedic wishes to administer diazepam to treat them, the paramedic may request assistance to hold/restrain the person for a few seconds so they can safely administer the drug: this is reasonable force. Conversely, if the person is injured as a result of being restrained then it could be argued that excessive rather than reasonable force was used.

Likewise, if the restraint method was inappropriate or prolonged, for example if the person was tied to the trolley or if they continued to be restrained after the drug had been administered, this would be considered unreasonable and therefore unlawful.

On the other hand, a person who becomes aggressive and displays threatening behaviour may require escalated restraint which may result in mild injuries such as bruising, due to the volatility of the situation. In such circumstances, it is vital that the least restrictive option is still adopted and restraint is relaxed as soon as it is safe to do so. Safety is always paramount, and the paramedic should feel confident that they will not sustain any injury themselves when restraining a person.

Deprivation of Liberty safeguards

Deprivation of Liberty safeguards (DoLS) apply in England and Wales – they were introduced in an amendment to MCA (2005).

The DoLS under the MCA (2005) allow restraint and restrictions that amount to a deprivation of liberty to be used in hospitals and care homes, but only if they are in a person's best interests. To deprive a person of their liberty, care homes and hospitals must request standard authorization in advance from a local authority.

Liberty Protection Safeguards (2018)

The Liberty Protection Safeguards (LPS) (2018) replace the DoL and broaden the scope to treat people, and deprive them of their liberty, in a medical emergency, without gaining prior authorization (Department of Health and Social Care 2021).

DoLs and LPS are not laws used by the paramedic, therefore they will not be discussed in detail in this chapter.

Human Rights Act 1998

After the Second World War, the Council of Europe was founded to protect human rights and the rule of law, and to promote democracy. The 47 member states drew up a treaty to secure basic rights for anyone within their borders, including their own citizens and people of other nationalities.

The European Convention on Human Rights (ECHR) consists of numbered 'articles' which protect the human rights of people in countries that belong to the Council of Europe.

The UK made these rights part of its domestic law through the Human Rights Act (1998), setting out the fundamental rights and freedoms that everyone in the UK is entitled to.

It is beyond the scope of this chapter to discuss every single article. The articles below have been selected as they are relevant to paramedic practice and mental health in the UK:

Article 2 – Right to life
Article 3 – Freedom from torture and inhuman or degrading treatment
Article 5 – Right to liberty and security
Article 8 – Right to respect for private and family life
Article 9 – Freedom of thought, conscience and religion
Article 14 – Protection from discrimination in respect of these rights and
freedoms

Table 2.7 Summary of Human Rights Act (1998)

Article	Some examples
2 – Right to Life Public authorities must: • not take away a person's life, except in a few very specific and very limited circumstances, such as lawfully, and using no more force than is absolutely necessary, defending someone from violence • take appropriate steps to protect a person's life in nearly all circumstances.	• Do not resuscitate orders • Active or passive euthanasia • Advance directives • Deaths through negligence • Investigations including inquests where a death is suspicious

(Continued)

Article	Some examples
3 – Freedom from torture and inhuman or degrading treatment • Inhuman treatment means treatment causing severe mental or physical suffering. • Degrading treatment means treatment that is grossly humiliating and undignified. • This is an absolute right.	• Physical or mental abuse • Failing to respect a person's dignity when conveying them to hospital – this includes a range of actions such as not covering them appropriately with a blanket, not cleaning a person if they have soiled themselves or indiscreetly handing over in a busy corridor • Excessive force used to restrain patients
5 – Right to liberty and security The right to liberty is a right not to be deprived of liberty in an arbitrary fashion. The right to liberty is a limited right. It can be limited in a number of specific circumstances, for example the lawful detention of someone who has mental health issues.	• Informal detention of patients who do not have the capacity to decide whether they would like to be admitted into hospital • Delays in reviewing whether mental health patients who are detained under the Mental Health Act should still be detained • Excessive restraint of patients, e.g. tying them to their beds or chairs for long periods
8 – Right to respect for private and family life This right can be split into four sections, which are the right to respect for: • private life – a person's privacy and body should not be invaded without their permission; this can include activities such as taking blood samples and performing body searches • family life – a person has the right to live with their family • one's home – a person has the right to live in their home in peace, without intrusion • correspondence – any type of correspondence such as letters, reports, emails etc. should be kept confidential and secure	• Family involvement in decision-making about a person's medical treatment – this must be balanced with respecting the person's confidentiality. • Any procedures that require physical contact, such as taking blood pressure or cannulation, should not be performed without the person's consent. • Assessing or examining a person can only be done with the person's consent. • Entering a person's home without permission from the home owner (e.g. s135). • A person's privacy should be respected in their own home. This means that a paramedic does not have the right to look in their cupboards or drawers (for medication, for example) without the person's consent. • Searching a person's bag or pockets. • Medical records and personal information must be kept confidential.

(Continued)

Table 2.7 (Continued)

Article	Some examples
9 – Freedom of thought, conscience and religion Different beliefs and religion can be held by the individual and are to be respected by others.	• Respect cultural and religious traditions or beliefs when a death has occurred. • Respect cultural and religious beliefs when assessing and treating an individual. For example, if a person requests a same-sex healthcare worker to treat them then this should be respected as far as is appropriate, providing it does not delay treatment in a time-critical incident.
14 – Protection from discrimination in respect of these rights and freedoms This right is a right not to be discriminated against in the enjoyment of the other human rights contained in the Human Rights Act. It is not a free-standing right, so if no other right in the Human Rights Act is engaged, then this right will not come into play. Discrimination takes place when someone is treated in a different way compared with someone else in a similar situation.	• Refusal of medical treatment to an older person solely because of their age (for example CPR). • Non-English speakers being presented with health options without the use of an interpreter.

Conclusion

Paramedics are tasked to deal with uncertainty as a major part of their role. The challenges posed while respecting a person's autonomy and acting in their best interests in the face of these uncertainties make it difficult for the paramedic to know what the best thing is to do. Ethical dilemmas and adherence to legal frameworks can be difficult to navigate as each individual situation demands different deliberations. Healthcare law regulates professional qualifications, ensures competent practice and protects the rights of service users. A basic understanding of ethical principles and healthcare law will help paramedics navigate through difficult dilemmas while providing person-centred care to the service user.

References

Adults with Incapacity (Scotland) Act 2000. Available at: https://www.legislation.gov.uk/asp/2000/4/contents (accessed 27 August 2020).

Augustus, J., Bold, J. and Williams, B. (2019) *An Introduction to Mental Health*. London: Sage.

Care Quality Commission (CQC) (2011) *The Mental Capacity Act 2005: Guidance for Providers*. Newcastle upon Tyne: CQC. Available at: https://www.cqc.org.uk/sites/default/files/documents/rp_poc1b2b_100563_20111223_v4_00_guidance_for_providers_mca_for_external_publication.pdf (accessed 27 August 2020).

Care Quality Commission (CQC) (2014) *A Safer Place to Be: Findings from our Survey of Health-Based Places of Safety for People Detained under section 136 of the Mental Health Act*. Newcastle upon Tyne: CQC. Available at: https://www.cqc.org.uk/sites/default/files/20141021%20CQC_SaferPlace_2014_07_FINAL%20for%20WEB.pdf (accessed 27 August 2020).

Department for Constitutional Affairs (2017) *Mental Capacity Act 2005: Code of Practice*. London: The Stationery Office. Available at: https://assets.publishing.service.gov.uk/government/uploads/system/uploads/attachment_data/file/497253/Mental-capacity-act-code-of-practice.pdf (accessed 27 August 2020).

Department of Health (DOH) (2015) *Mental Health Act: Code of Practice*. London: The Stationery Office. Available at: https://assets.publishing.service.gov.uk/government/uploads/system/uploads/attachment_data/file/435512/MHA_Code_of_Practice.PDF (accessed 27 August 2020).

Department of Health (DOH) (2017) *Guidance for the Implementation of Changes to Police Powers and Places of Safety Provisions in the Mental Health Act 1983*. Available at: https://assets.publishing.service.gov.uk/government/uploads/system/uploads/attachment_data/file/656025/Guidance_on_Police_Powers.PDF (accessed 27 August 2020).

Department of Health (DOH) (2018) *Modernising the Mental Health Act – Final Report from the Independent Review*. Available at: https://www.gov.uk/government/publications/modernising-the-mental-health-act-final-report-from-the-independent-review (accessed 1 July 2021).

Department of Health (DOH) (2019) *Deprivation of Liberty Safeguards: Code of Practice*. Belfast: Department of Health. Available at: https://www.health-ni.gov.uk/sites/default/files/publications/health/mca-dols-cop-november-2019.pdf (accessed 26 June 2021).

Department of Health and Social Care (2017) *Five Year Forward View for Mental Health: Government Response*. Available at: https://www.gov.uk/government/publications/five-year-forward-view-for-mental-health-government-response (accessed 1 July 2021).

Department of Health and Social Care (2021) Liberty Protection Safeguards. Available at: https://www.gov.uk/government/publications/liberty-protection-safeguards-factsheets/liberty-protection-safeguards-what-they-are (accessed 19 August 2021).

Human Rights Act 1998. Available at: https://www.legislation.gov.uk/ukpga/1998/42/contents (accessed 27 August 2020).

Jacobsen, P., Hodkinson, K., Peters, E. and Chadwick, P. (2018) A systematic scoping review of psychological therapies for psychosis within acute psychiatric in-patient settings, *British Journal of Psychiatry*, 213(2): 490–7.

Mental Capacity Act 2005. Available at: https://www.legislation.gov.uk/ukpga/2005/9/contents (accessed: 27 August 2020)

Mental Capacity Act Code of Practice 2013. Available at: https://www.gov.uk/government/publications/mental-capacity-act-code-of-practice (accessed 27 August 2020).

Mental Capacity Act (Northern Ireland) (2016). Available at: https://www.legislation.gov.uk/nia/2016/18/contents/enacted (accessed 18 August 2021).

Mental Health Act 1983. Available at: https://www.legislation.gov.uk/ukpga/1983/20/contents (accessed 27 August 2020).

Mental Health Act 2007. Available at: https://www.legislation.gov.uk/ukpga/2007/12/contents (accessed 27 August 2020).

Mental Health (Care and Treatment) (Scotland) Act 2003. Available at: https://www.legislation.gov.uk/asp/2003/13/contents (accessed 27 August 2020).

Mental Health (Northern Ireland) Order (1986). Available at: https://www.legislation.gov.uk/nisi/1986/595 (accessed 18 August 2021).

Mental Health (Scotland) Act (2015). Available at: https://www.legislation.gov.uk/asp/2015/9/contents (accessed 18 August 2021).

National Institute for Health and Care Excellence (NICE) (2009) *Borderline Personality Disorder: Recognition and Management.* Clinical guideline CG78. Available at: https://www.nice.org.uk/guidance/cg78 (accessed 28 May 2021).

National Institute for Health and Care Excellence (NICE) (2014) *Psychosis and Schizophrenia in Adults: Prevention and Management.* Clinical guideline CG178. Available at: https://www.nice.org.uk/guidance/cg178 (accessed 13 August 2021).

Paterson, C., Karatzias, T., Dickson, A., Harper, S., Dougall, N. and Hutton, P. (2018) Psychological therapy for inpatients receiving acute mental health care: A systematic review and meta-analysis of controlled trials, *British Journal of Clinical Psychology*, 57(4): 453–72.

Skills for Care and Skills for Health (2014) *A Positive and Proactive Workforce. A Guide to Workforce Development for Commissioners and Employers seeking to Minimise the use of Restrictive Practices in Social Care and Health.* Leeds: Skills for Care / Bristol: Skills for Health. Available at: https://www.skillsforcare.org.uk/Documents/Topics/Restrictive-practices/A-positive-and-proactive-workforce.pdf (accessed 27 August 2020).

Sustere, E. and Tarpey, E. (2019) Least restrictive practice: Its role in patient independence and recovery, *Journal of Forensic Psychiatry and Psychology*, 30(4): 614–29.

The Royal College of Emergency Medicine (RCEM) (2017) *A Brief Guide to Section 136 for Emergency Departments.* London: RCEM. Available at: https://www.rcem.ac.uk/docs/College%20Guidelines/A%20brief%20guide%20to%20Section%20136%20for%20Emergency%20Departments%20-%20Dec%202017.pdf (accessed 27 August 2020).

Wood, L., Williams, C., Billings, J. and Johnson, S. (2019) Psychologists' perspectives on the implementation of psychological therapy for psychosis in the acute psychiatric inpatient setting, *Qualitative Health Research*, 29(14): 2048–56.

3 How mental health conditions can develop

Paula Gardner

Learning objectives

- Consider risk factors for developing mental health conditions
- Look at bio-psycho-social aspects to mental health
- Explore adverse childhood experiences (ACEs) and the link between ACEs and the development of mental health conditions in adulthood
- Discuss internal and external risk factors for developing a mental health condition
- Consider the impact of the COVID-19 pandemic on mental health

Introduction

Everyone experiences challenges in their lives, and in times of difficulty feeling negative emotions such as anger or low mood, or having difficulty sleeping is often a natural response when dealing with stressful situations. There is no 'right' or 'wrong' way to react and some people can be more intensely affected by certain events than others.

There are several factors that can affect mental health, which include internal factors such as the ability to manage our thoughts, emotions, behaviours and relationships with others, and external factors such as social, cultural, economic and political. Personal or work-related stress, genetics, life experiences, nutritional health, perinatal infections and environmental factors are also thought to contribute to the development of mental health conditions. Although many of these factors, including occupation, diet, drugs and alcohol and interruption to normal sleep patterns, can all negatively affect mental health, mental health conditions often develop due to a combination of factors and may depend on the amount of support a person has around them at the time (MIND 2017; Augustus et al. 2019). A mental health condition is a continuation of debilitating symptoms which is often termed severe and enduring mental illness. (See Chapter 4 for further information on common mental health conditions.)

Information box 3.1   Bio-psycho-social model in mental health

The bio-psycho-social model was developed by Engel in 1980 to identify the links between biological and psychological needs that had been traditionally treated independently of each other. The model recognizes that social, psychological and biological factors influence each other, and the three elements of health have a combined influence on efficacy of treatment, as mental illness is often associated with comorbidities from a wide range of physical health conditions (Watters and Martin 2021).

Risk factors for poor mental health

There are a number of factors which can influence mental health, including:

- Adverse childhood experiences (ACEs) such as childhood abuse, trauma or neglect
- Being socially isolated
- Suffering from discrimination
- Financial issues such as debt
- Bereavement, suffering the loss of a loved one
- Extreme stress – personal or work-related
- Chronic or long-term medical conditions or a terminal diagnosis
- Unemployment
- Changing jobs or schools
- Homelessness
- Divorce
- Caring for someone who has a medical condition
- Substance misuse (by the person or their carers) – long-term substance use has been linked to anxiety, depression and feelings of paranoia
- Experiencing domestic violence, bullying or harassment
- Feelings of inadequacy, low self-esteem or loneliness
- Social or cultural expectations – e.g. media influences such as 'size zero' models can lead to the development of eating disorders
- Traumatic events such as military combat or being involved in a serious life-threatening incident
- Neurological causes such as traumatic brain injury (TBI) or a condition such as epilepsy which can alter mood and behaviour
- Infections – certain infections have been linked to brain damage and the development of mental health conditions or exacerbation of symptoms – a condition known as paediatric autoimmune neuropsychiatric disorder associated with the streptococcus bacteria has been linked to the development of obsessive-compulsive disorder and other mental health conditions in children
- Prenatal damage – there is evidence to suggest that a disruption of early foetal brain development, or trauma that occurs at the time of birth such as hypoxia, may be a factor in the development of certain conditions such as autism spectrum disorder
- Other factors – dysfunctional upbringing, poor nutrition and exposure to environmental toxins such as lead

(Adapted from MIND 2017; Augustus et al. 2019)

Genetics and mental health

Research around genetics and mental health has shown that certain mental health conditions such as schizophrenia, bipolar disorder, anxiety, depression and obsessive-compulsive disorder (OCD) may run in families, suggesting that people who have a family member with a mental health condition may be potentially more likely to develop one themselves. However, it is not known if this is due to genetics or because of behaviours learnt from parents during childhood. While some mental health conditions are potentially influenced by genetics, there are many people who develop mental health conditions where there are no other relatives in the family with the same condition.

Genetically inherited disorders are acquired as a result of autosomal genetic mutations that are either present at birth or are developed during the life course. Environmental factors play a key role in the development of mental health conditions, and where several genes interact with these factors it may increase the likelihood of developing a disorder, but it is not thought to be a direct cause (Blows 2016). Experts believe that many mental health conditions are linked to abnormalities in many genes rather than just one or a few, and that how these genes interact with the environment is unique for every person.

Therefore, a person who inherits a susceptibility to a mental health condition doesn't necessarily develop the illness. The mental health condition itself occurs from the interaction of multiple genes and other factors – such as stress, abuse or a traumatic event – which can influence, or trigger, an illness in a person who has an inherited susceptibility to it (Kinsella and Kinsella 2015; Augustus et al. 2019).

Neurotransmitters

Research has shown that mental health conditions can arise due to a problem with the communication between the neurons in the brain (neurotransmission). For example, serotonin levels have been found to be lower in people who have depression. Selective serotonin reuptake inhibitors (SSRIs) work by reducing the amount of serotonin that is taken back into the presynaptic neuron, which increases the amount of serotonin present in the synaptic space for binding to the receptor on the postsynaptic neuron. Changes in serotonin and other neurotransmitters may occur in depression, which adds to the complexity of the treatment of the underlying condition (see Chapter 6 for further information on commonly prescribed medications).

Serotonin – known as the 'mood hormone', serotonin regulates sleep, is linked to memory and is involved in peristalsis. It is thought to be involved in feelings of ecstasy but also leads to an increased risk of suicide, which is controversial given the prescribing of antidepressants which increase serotonin levels.

Dopamine – involved in coordination and body movement as well as cognitive functions such as attention and problem solving. In patients with Parkinson's, the brain is unable to produce sufficient levels of dopamine, leading to issues in communication between the brain and the musculoskeletal system which cause the tremor associated with parkinsonian symptoms. Illicit drugs such as cocaine act on dopamine receptors, which results in a euphoric feeling. Excessive dopamine is linked to psychosis; treatments such as antipsychotic medication block the action and reduce symptoms.

Noradrenaline – involved in the 'fight or flight' response, noradrenaline regulates mood and is thought to be linked with cognitive processes such as motivation and reward (Kinsella and Kinsella 2015). As with reduced serotonin, low levels of noradrenaline are associated with depression and low mood.

Glutamate – found in large quantities in the brain, glutamate has recently been discovered as a potential factor in the onset of psychosis, particularly when combined with overproduction of dopamine (Kinsella and Kinsella 2015).

Adverse childhood experiences and mental health

There is growing evidence which suggests that experiencing traumatic events in childhood increases the susceptibility of developing mental health conditions such as depression, post-traumatic stress disorder (PTSD), personality disorder, substance misuse and psychosis (Tew and BASW 2011). Adverse childhood experiences (ACEs) can have profound and long-lasting effects on physical and mental health, and a greater number of ACEs experienced is associated with a higher risk of adverse health outcomes (Bomysoad and Francis 2020). ACEs include household dysfunction, neglect, physical and sexual abuse, or trauma such as the loss of a parent, and are associated with increased risk of negative mental and physical health outcomes and early mortality (Schalinski et al. 2016).

Studies conducted on adverse childhood experiences have revealed some interesting links between ACEs and impairment of brain structure and function due to increased exposure of the developing brain to stressor responses. Morphological changes in brain structures such as the prefrontal cortex (responsible for attention, executive function and self-regulation) and hippocampus (responsible for emotion), functional changes such as enhanced amygdala response to emotional facial expressions and alterations in grey matter volume have been found in participants who experienced extreme parental verbal abuse as a child (Navalta et al. 2018). Bryan (2019) also states that ACEs can have a profound effect on the developing brain as neurons function based on repeated experiences, and the brains of children growing up in toxic situations function out of survival mode.

Zhang et al. (2021) explored converging evidence from research in foetal development and maternal adverse childhood experiences, such as physical, emotional or sexual abuse and neglect, and found an association with long-term impact on emotional, cognitive and behavioural outcomes, with an increased risk of mental health conditions in the offspring. Children of mothers with depression experience similar developmental outcomes as well as an increased risk of childhood maltreatment or depression, and often have similar psychological problems and brain abnormalities in the frontal, temporal and sensory regions, which may suggest an inheritance of these conditions across the generations.

Bryan (2019) believes that healthcare professionals with an understanding of ACEs in a primary care setting should practise trauma-informed care to explore what has happened to a patient, as opposed to what is wrong with them, in order to understand their behaviour. Creating a safe environment, respecting privacy and allowing loved ones to be present during assessment may encourage the patient to disclose adverse childhood experiences. This allows the healthcare professional to recognize the prevalence and effect of the exposure on health and well-being, creating a shift in perspective that has the potential to increase empathy and compassion in our patient care.

Dementia and depression

There are approximately 50 million people globally who have been diagnosed with a form of dementia, with a rapidly increasing rate of incidence (Ali et al. 2015; WHO 2019). Dementia is a chronic and progressive condition in which there is a deterioration in cognition which can severely impact activities of daily living, and can be caused by disease or injury affecting the brain, such as Alzheimer's disease or cerebrovascular accident (CVA) (WHO 2019). Current research has shown that there are links between dementia and depression, with some studies showing depression as a symptom of dementia and other studies that show depression as a possible cause of dementia (Nasisi 2020). Risk factors associated with the development of Alzheimer's disease are thought to be diabetes, hypertension, obesity, reduced exercise, depression, smoking and lack of education (Norton et al. 2014). Nasisi (2020) believes that it is important for clinicians to be aware of the psychosocial risk factors for dementia, including depression, isolation and stress, in order to help prevent the disease.

Long-term health conditions

A long-term condition, or chronic illness, is a term used to describe any ongoing health condition that can be managed but not cured, which can impact on daily life and requires self-management of symptoms and/or treatments (Wilson and Stock 2019).

There is clear evidence of the interrelationship between physical and mental health conditions – in some cases mental health conditions can impact on the severity of a physical health condition, reducing quality of life and leading to poorer patient outcomes (Naylor 2013). Conditions such as asthma, epilepsy, cerebral palsy, arthritis and cystic fibrosis have all been linked to mental health conditions such as anxiety and depression. Young adults living with long-term conditions have reported feelings of low mood, depression, suicidal thoughts, anxiety, fear for the future and difficulty accepting their condition (Wilson and Stock 2019). Conditions which cause pain and sleep deprivation in children have been associated with behavioural problems, social isolation and attention deficit hyperactivity disorder (ADHD) (Whitney et al. 2019).

Management of the psychosocial consequences of a long-term condition is thought to be an important aspect of patient care to help improve clinical outcomes (Catanzano et al. 2020). Paramedics regularly attend patients with long-term conditions who have called due to an exacerbation of a chronic illness or a sudden onset of an acute problem (Abrashkin et al. 2016), therefore it is important to understand the risk factors for potential underlying mental health conditions that are associated with this patient group.

Older adults living in long-term care

Older adults living in long-term care are around four times more likely to develop depression than older adults who live in their own home, but despite the high prevalence it is largely under-diagnosed and under-treated (Jongenelis et al. 2004). The links between depression in older adults and increased mortality and comorbidity, physical and mental health decline, risk of suicide, greater reliance on personal care and health services, and reduced quality of life highlight the importance of managing depression in residents living in long-term care settings (Davison et al. 2018).

Most clinicians in their daily practice will encounter older patients with depression. Physical factors such as long-term conditions, chronic pain, social isolation, change in financial status (losing their home to pay for care), loss of social status and difficulty in adapting to a new environment can increase the risk of depression (Rodda et al. 2011). Jongenelis et al. (2004) believe that residents who suffer with pain, visual impairment and have a history of stroke are at greater risk of developing mental health conditions. Psychosocial factors such as loneliness or isolation, recent adverse life events (such as loss of a spouse), lack of social support and feelings of inadequate care can all lead to depression in residents in long-term care (Brennan and SooHoo 2020).

Caring for someone with support needs

Carers are those who provide care and support for someone who is unable to independently care for themselves and their own needs due to a chronic illness, disability, frailty or a mental health condition, and are often family members or friends who do not receive any pay (Augustus et al. 2019).

Those who care for family members experience a variety of challenges such as lack of access to community services, financial difficulties often associated with loss of income or having to give up or reduce paid employment, and lack of recognition among healthcare professionals. They also report adverse physical, emotional and social outcomes due to their role as caregiver (Teahan et al. 2021).

Research in carers of children with cancer have highlighted the prevalence of mental health problems which affect parents, siblings and the wider family due to coming to terms with the diagnosis, carer conflict, anticipatory grief and financial concerns (Elliott et al. 2021). The mental health problems experienced can have an impact on the child's medical treatment, parenting of the ill child and any siblings, and can disrupt usual family functioning. Elliott et al. (2021) emphasize the importance of early and continuing assessment and support of the mental health needs of the caregivers and siblings of children with cancer.

As a paramedic it is important to ensure the well-being of patients and their carers, and 'encourage and help service users, where appropriate, to maintain their own health and well-being, and support them so they can make informed decisions' (HCPC 2016).

The COVID-19 pandemic and the impact on mental health

The COVID-19 pandemic caused a dramatic risk to public health globally and has had a huge socio-economic impact, particularly associated with the restrictive and confining measures imposed to contain the disease, raising concerns about an emerging international mental health crisis (Dos Santos et al. 2020). Lockdowns resulted in a huge and rapid alteration to normal life, with sudden separation from loved ones, shortages in living supplies, and financial concerns due to job redundancies or reduction in salaries (Chen et al. 2020).

Shah (2020) highlights the association with exposure to disasters and the risk of developing mental health conditions such as post-traumatic stress disorder (PTSD), major depressive disorder (MDD), substance use, anxiety and panic disorders, phobias and neuropsychiatric disorders, and also warns of the risk of prolonged isolation on the prevalence of domestic violence and child abuse. This viewpoint is supported by early studies on the impact on the mental health of vulnerable groups such as healthcare workers, which found that the pandemic has resulted in stress, anxiety and depression, and an increased risk in the use of substances, suicide, domestic violence and complicated grief (Dos Santos et al. 2020).

Previous epidemics, such as Influenza A (H1N1), have shown correlations between emotional distress (such as anxiety and depression) and viral diseases, and it is anticipated that the social isolation, lack of peer-supported learning and educational disruptions that have ensued from COVID-19 might also influence children and adolescents' future mental health.

Conclusion

This chapter has explored some of the risk factors associated with the development of a mental health condition and has highlighted that anyone is at risk of developing a mental health condition at any point in their lives. It is important that paramedics have an awareness of the risk factors and recognize the patient groups who may be more susceptible to developing a severe and enduring mental health condition. Risk factors can be internal or external, modifiable or non-modifiable, and there is often a combination of factors which results in the onset of a mental health condition. Support networks are incredibly important and should be explored with patients who may be identified as experiencing or at risk of experiencing a mental health condition.

At the time of writing this chapter, research is ongoing into the global implications of the COVID-19 pandemic for mental health, and the extent of the bio-psycho-social impact may not be understood for some time.

References

Abrashkin, K.A., Washko, J., Zhang, J., Poku, A., Kim, H. and Smith, K.L. (2016) Providing acute care at home: Community paramedics enhance an advanced illness management program – preliminary data, *Journal of the American Geriatrics Society (JAGS)*, 64(12): 2572–6.

Ali, G.C., Guerchet, M., Yu-Tzu, W., Prince, M. and Prina, M. (2015) The global prevalence of dementia, in M. Prince et al. (eds) *World Alzheimer Report 2015: The Global Impact of Dementia*. London: Alzheimer's Disease International, pp. 10–29.

Augustus, J., Bold, J. and Williams, B. (2019) *An Introduction to Mental Health*. London: SAGE.

Blows, W.T. (2016) *The Biological Basis of Mental Health*, 3rd edn. London: Routledge.

Bomysoad, R.N. and Francis, L.A. (2020) Adverse childhood experiences and mental health conditions among adolescents, *Journal of Adolescent Health*, 67(6): 868–70.

Brennan, P.L. and SooHoo, S. (2020) Effects of mental health disorders on nursing home residents' nine-month pain trajectories, *Pain Medicine*, 21(3): 488–500.

Bryan, R.H. (2019) Getting to why: Adverse childhood experiences' impact on adult health, *Journal for Nurse Practitioners*, 15(2) 153–7.e1.

Catanzano, M., Bennett, S.D., Sanderson, C. et al. (2020) Brief psychological interventions for psychiatric disorders in young people with long term physical health conditions: A systematic review and meta-analysis, *Journal of Psychosomatic Research*, 136(4): 110187.

Chen, S., Cheng, Z. and Wu, J. (2020) Risk factors for adolescents' mental health during the COVID-19 pandemic: A comparison between Wuhan and other urban areas in China, *Globalization and Health*, 16(1): 96.

Davison, T.E., You, E., Doyle, C., Bhar, S., Wells, Y. and Flicker, L. (2018) Psychological therapies for depression in older adults residing in long-term care settings, *Cochrane Library Database of Systematic Reviews*, 6. doi: 10.1002/14651858.CD013059.

Dos Santos, C.F., Pica-Perez, M. and Morgado, P. (2020) COVID-19 and mental health – what do we know so far?, *Frontiers in Psychiatry*, 11: 565698.

Elliott, D.A., Corneau-Dia, D.E., Turner, E., Barnett, B. and Parris, K.R. (2021) Caregiver mental health in paediatric oncology: A three-tiered model of supports, *Psycho-Oncology*, 30(2): 267–70.

Health and Care Professions Council (HCPC) (2016) *Standards of Conduct, Performance and Ethics*, HPCP website. Available at: https://www.hcpc-uk.org/standards/standards-of-conduct-performance-and-ethics/ (accessed 3 June 2021).

Jongenelis, K., Pot, A.M., Eisses, A.M.H., Beekman, A.T.F., Kluiter, H. and Ribbe, M.W. (2004) Prevalence and risk indicators of depression in elderly nursing home patients: The AGED study, *Journal of Affective Disorders*, 83(2–3): 135–42.

Kinsella, C. and Kinsella, C. (2015) *Introducing Mental Health: A Practical Guide*, 2nd edn. London: Jessica Kingsley Publishers.

MIND (2017) *Mental Health Problems – An Introduction*, MIND website. Available at: https://www.mind.org.uk/information-support/types-of-mental-health-problems/mental-health-problems-introduction/causes/ (accessed 25 May 2021).

Nasisi, C.R. (2020) Dementia: Psychosocial/mental health risk factors, *Journal for Nurse Practitioners*, 16(6): 425–7.

Navalta, C.P., McGee, L. and Underwood, J. (2018) Adverse childhood experiences, brain development, and mental health: A call for neurocounseling, *Journal of Mental Health Counseling*, 40(3): 266–78.

Naylor, C. (2013) SP0115 The link between long-term conditions and mental health, *Annals of the Rheumatic Diseases*, 71(Supp3): 28–9.

Norton, S., Matthews, F.E., Barnes, D.E., Yaffe, K. and Brayne, C. (2014) Potential for primary prevention of Alzheimer's disease: An analysis of population-based data, *Lancet Neurology*, 13(8): 788–94.

Rodda, J., Walker, Z. and Carter, J. (2011) Depression in older adults, *BMJ*, 343(7825). doi: 10.1136/bmj.d5219.

Schalinski, I., Teicher, M.H., Nischk, D., Hinderer, E., Müller, O. and Rockstroh, B. (2016) Type and timing of adverse childhood experiences differentially affect severity of PTSD, dissociative and depressive symptoms in adult inpatients, *BMC Psychiatry*, 16: 295.

Shah, A.A. (2020) COVID-19 and Mental Health, *Psychiatric Annals*, 50(12): 519–20.

Teahan, Á., Lafferty, A., Cullinan, J., Fealy, G. and O'Shea, E. (2021) An analysis of carer burden among family carers of people with and without dementia in Ireland, *International Psychogeriatrics*, 33(4): 347–58.

Tew, J. and British Association of Social Workers (2011) *Social Approaches to Mental Distress*. Basingstoke: Palgrave Macmillan.

Watters, E.R. and Martin, G. (2021) Health outcomes following childhood maltreatment: An examination of the biopsychosocial model, *Journal of Aging and Health*, 33(7–8): 596–606. doi: 10.1177/08982643211003783.

Whitney, D.G., Warschausky, S.A. and Peterson, M.D. (2019) Mental health disorders and physical risk factors in children with cerebral palsy: A cross-sectional study, *Developmental Medicine and Child Neurology*, 61(5): 579-585.

Wilson, C. and Stock, J. (2019) The impact of living with long-term conditions in young adulthood on mental health and identity: What can help?, *Health Expectations: An International Journal of Public Participation in Health Care and Health Policy*, 22(5): 1111–21.

World Health Organization (WHO) (2019) *Mental Disorders*, WHO website. Available at: https://www.who.int/news-room/fact-sheets/detail/mental-disorders (accessed 2 June 2021).

Zhang, H., Wong, T., Broekman, B.F.P. et al. (2021) Maternal adverse childhood experience and depression in relation with brain network development and behaviors in children: A longitudinal study, *Cerebral Cortex*, 31(9): 4233–44. doi: 10.1093/cercor/bhab081.

4 Mental health diagnoses

Jo Augustus

Learning objectives

- Consider the types of diagnostic criteria used by mental health professionals
- Explore different types of mental health conditions and their key characteristics
- Consider the interaction of mental health and physical health
- Discuss the contested position of mental health diagnosis and the implications for pre-hospital care

Introduction

Effective pre-hospital care requires a working knowledge of diagnostic criteria. It is widely recognized that there are two classification systems that are used in routine clinical practice to diagnose psychiatric conditions: firstly, the International Classification of Diseases system (ICD), published by the World Health Organization (WHO), and secondly, the Diagnostic and Statistical Manual of Mental Disorders (DSM), published by the American Psychiatric Association. These are regularly updated to reflect current research and as such often see significant changes in the way diagnoses are presented. It is therefore important to use the most recently published version – at the time of writing, ICD-11 or version 11 and DSM-V or version five are both in operation.

This chapter will explore both the context and the relevance of DSM-V and ICD-11 to clinical practice, including the history of diagnostic criteria, the assessment process and the context of this for the actual diagnosis of anxiety and mood disorders. It will set out the key characteristics of both common and severe and enduring mental health difficulties. The contested nature of mental health diagnoses will also be considered, as well as how this can lead to misdiagnosis.

Why is diagnostic criteria relevant to paramedics?

This chapter is exploring different diagnoses relevant to emergency medicine: let's take a step back and consider why mental health diagnostic criteria is relevant to paramedicine. DSM and ICD provide current diagnostic criteria relevant to each disorder for clinicians to apply in practice. This offers a standardized approach, meaning that care is provided consistently, and arguably in an evidence-based way. Therefore, an individual being treated in two different geographical locations in the UK will receive similar treatment on their path to recovery. But it's important to acknowledge that there are geographical variations in the way services are operated, so recovery may differ. Diagnostic criteria also account for sociocultural change, therefore diagnostic criteria ensure clinical practice is inclusive, appropriate and reflective of advancements made. The demand for ambulance services has grown and there is evidence to suggest that those individuals with comorbidity specific to mental health access the health service more frequently (Rolfe et al. 2020). This may include an individual experiencing an acute episode, for instance a failed suicide attempt or deliberate self-harm. As paramedics are often the first to respond it is essential they have a working knowledge of diagnostic criteria in order to respond to the pre-hospital care needs of their patients.

A short history of mental health diagnostics

The very first ICD, in 1893, identified an International List of Causes of Death. Upon its creation the WHO became involved from 1948. The first DSM was published in 1952 using information collated over a 60-year period, with specific reference to the identified needs of active service personnel involved in the Second World War. DSM-I therefore saw initial attempts to construct diagnostic criteria for use in the military, and DSM-II was published in 1968 following research in the post-war period. Around this time clinicians started evaluating DSM-II, acknowledging some of the disadvantages of its application to clinical practice and its reliability. Subsequently, there was an acknowledgement that diagnostic criteria could lead clinicians to provide different diagnoses for the same symptoms. The two later versions were amended, with DSM-III published in 1980 and DSM-IV in 1994, which provided more accessible information, detailing how diagnostic criteria had to be met. DSM-V, published in 2013, has produced subsets of disorders, which enables further refinement of the diagnosis. These revisions have been met with much controversy, as, in short, including diagnoses that arguably could be part of everyday life such as depression following a bereavement. In summary, the DSM has developed over time to provide clinicians with a comprehensive guide (Augustus et al. 2019).

What is the difference between ICD-11 and DSM-V?: classification systems

ICD-11

ICD-11 was developed by the WHO to provide a means for standardizing diagnostic criteria for the management of health and mental health (WHO 2018). A central function is to collate and share statistical information about morbidity and mortality. This enables comparisons of statistical information at a global level and reliable cross-cultural application to clinical practice. It is updated periodically and published free online.

DSM-V

DSM-V was developed by the American Psychiatric Association and is used predominantly in America, although its use is promoted globally. It provides standardized criteria in the classification of mental health difficulties. The impact of a mental health difficulty is acknowledged, such as the distress caused by disruption to an individual's cognitive, emotional or behavioural patterns. DSM is regularly updated and it encourages its users to see it as a working document that responds to change.

There are both similarities and differences between DSM-V and ICD-11, summarized in Table 4.1.

Table 4.1 A summary comparison of ICD and DSM

ICD	DSM
Compiled by an international organization	Compiled by a national organization
Freely available online	A resource that has to be purchased
Includes mental and physical health	Includes mental health only
Adopts a global perspective	Largely an American perspective
Aimed at all clinicians	Aimed largely at psychiatrists

Why have diagnostic criteria?

Throughout history the sciences have used classification systems as a way to present the foundations of their subject. Thus, these systems offer ways to understand the information an individual is presenting – e.g. verbal or non-verbal. We can then use this information to consider causation (also known as triggers) as part of the triage assessment. However, it is important to remember the cause is only one factor; the paramedic would also need to establish additional aspects, such as physical observations, current risk of threat to life and maintenance factors. Therefore, while they are important, classification systems are just one component of the wider paramedic assessment process.

What are some of the difficulties with diagnosis?

Pause for thought

As you read the case study, consider:

What might be some of the challenges that Kelly has faced? Hint: consider the impact of having more than one diagnosis.

Case study 4.1 Personality disorder

Kelly (28 years old) has been detained under the Mental Health Act on many occasions, for both assessment and treatment since she was 18 years old, although her mental health difficulties stem back to the age of 12 years. Aged 12, Kelly was sexually abused by an older man over a three-year period, which ended when he was charged and imprisoned.

Kelly developed various inappropriate friendships and relationships with people much older than herself. She began to binge drink alcohol, smoke, and occasionally used non-prescription drugs to fit into her social group. Her attendance at school was erratic, and aged 16 years she was excluded from school due to her physically and verbally abusive behaviour towards staff. She left home and began sleeping rough for periods of time, before returning home. It was during this time that Kelly began to develop maladaptive coping strategies, including cutting herself. Kelly stopped eating regularly, she developed insomnia, she didn't get out of bed for days at a time and began hallucinating. The emergency services were called on various occasions to her home and to areas where she socialized, typically the local pubs. This often resulted from her consuming alcohol and/or drugs, arguing with her boyfriend and then threatening to kill herself if he left her. On occasion she cut herself with a sharp object to different degrees of severity, leading to the emergency services being called.

After assessing Kelly the emergency service involvement often resulted in her being taken to a place of safety or A&E department, where she was further assessed and on occasion detained under the Mental Health Act. This led to long stays in her local inpatient mental health unit. During her various admissions to hospital she was given different diagnoses that included: depression, anorexia, bipolar disorder with psychosis. On her most recent admission a psychiatrist diagnosed her with a personality disorder.

> **Information box 4.1 What are maladaptive coping strategies?**
>
> These can be seen as unhealthy coping strategies, often attempting to deal with stressful events, such as avoidance, denial or a behaviour that results in self-harm. It is recognized that these coping strategies often develop in childhood, often in response to adverse childhood experiences. More recently emphasis has been placed on reframing these coping styles as functional adaptations (Wadsworth 2015).

Different types of mental health difficulties

Once a diagnosis has been outlined, consideration can then be given to a pathway of care. The National Institute for Clinical Excellence (NICE) has developed guidance on both identification and care pathways. Therefore, NICE guidelines shift away from purely focusing on the diagnoses and consider evidence-based interventions. The following will consider two broad categories of mental health difficulties: common mental health problems, and severe and enduring mental health problems. It is not an exhaustive list; rather it aims to highlight mental health difficulties that paramedics are expected to encounter. The reader will be signposted to further reading as appropriate, should they wish to explore a particular diagnosis in more detail.

As their titles suggest, the former considers symptoms as short term with a lower impact, and the latter indicates long-term symptoms with significant impact on an individual's functioning. Thus, longevity of symptoms and the impact these symptoms have on an individual's day-to-day functioning are central considerations. Although it is important to note that an individual's symptoms can be changeable – in other words they could become severe, or indeed have a more limited impact on daily functioning. Equally, some common mental health problems can be debilitating and have a significant impact on the individual, while some symptoms associated with severe and enduring mental health difficulties could have a minimal impact on functioning. Therefore, such categories could be viewed as being too reductionist, meaning they are looking at the individual symptoms rather than taking a whole person approach. A whole person approach is central to person-centred care, the cornerstone of healthcare. As an extreme consequence, this could lead to misdiagnosis and therefore the wrong treatment plan. As such, the reader is encouraged to see these as broad categories that are used to gain a general understanding of the presenting symptoms.

Information box 4.2 Diagnosis: children and young people

The World Health Organization reported an estimated 10–20 per cent of children and young people (CYP) as experiencing a mental health difficulty before reaching adulthood (Kessler et al. 2007; WHO 2020). Cohen et al. (2020) reported that symptoms associated with severe and enduring mental health difficulties typically start before age 25. Research has indicated that mental health conditions that begin during childhood increase the likelihood of developing mental health problems in adulthood (Cohen et al. 2020). For example, attention deficit hyperactivity disorder (ADHD) in CYP is a predictor of bipolar disorder in adulthood (Biederman et al. 2009; Duffy 2012; Duffy et al. 2014). Thus, early intervention is essential to prevent the deterioration of symptoms. However, Waid and Kelly (2020) have identified various barriers to accessing appropriate services in a timely way. Duong et al. (2021) reported that more than 25 per cent of children and young people with a mental health diagnosis or who were experiencing mental health symptoms were not accessing mental health services. This indicates that the accessibility of mental health services for CYP needs to be reviewed, to overcome the identified barriers and improve access. In addition, this may indicate that children and families may be increasingly accessing pre-hospital care. Therefore, paramedics may also increasingly encounter difficulties associated with CYP mental health, especially those in crisis (Banwell et al. 2021).

Mental health diagnoses

This section will move on to explore individual diagnoses. In order to help the reader to link these to practice, the following structure will be adopted.

- Symptoms and signs – including an exploration of causes and characteristics
- Impact on the individual, family and friends – including any change of role and responsibilities
- Where misdiagnosis can occur – including the overlap between some medical diagnoses and different mental health difficulties
- Care pathway – including the interventions that may be received after pre-hospital care
- A line of questioning that could be adopted – including questions to aid the paramedic assessment as part of providing patient-centred care

NICE identified the following common mental health problems, summarized in Table 4.2 (NICE 2011).

Table 4.2 A summary of common mental health problems

Depression	Obsessive-compulsive disorder (OCD)
Generalized anxiety disorder (GAD)	Post-traumatic stress disorder (PTSD)
Panic disorder	Simple phobias

Adapted from NICE (2011) and Kendrick and Pilling (2012)

Anxiety disorders

Anxiety could be seen as a normal reaction to stress and it can be beneficial as an alert to danger and subsequently help us prepare and/or pay attention. However, anxiety disorders involve excessive fear or anxiety and therefore can be differentiated from what we may term normal feelings of anxiousness. In general, for a person to be diagnosed with an anxiety disorder, the fear or anxiety must:

• be out of proportion to the situation or age-inappropriate
• hinder your ability to function normally

Anxiety usually refers to worries related to anticipation of the future, and is usually typified by physical response, such as increased breathing or muscle tension, and associated avoidance behaviours. The presence of fear is often noted, frequently depicted by the flight, fight or freeze response as an emotional response to a perceived immediate threat. As a result, anxiety disorders can have a significant impact on day-to-day functioning, including, but not limited to, job, education and relationships. The following is not an exhaustive list, however it seeks to summarize some of the more common anxiety disorders.

Generalized anxiety disorder

Generalized anxiety disorder (GAD) is typified by excessive anxiety and worry: the notion of apprehensive expectation or what is sometimes noted as free-floating anxiety. It is expected to have been persistent for several months, occurring on more days than not (WHO 2018). A person with GAD finds it difficult to control the anxiety and worry, which frequently concern family, health, finances and education or workplace. This is often accompanied by motor restlessness, being easily fatigued, difficulty concentrating, irritability, muscle tension and sleep disturbance (Brown et al. 2001). The symptoms often lead to significant distress or impairment in personal, family, social, educational, occupational or other important areas of functioning.

Some people with GAD may become excessively apprehensive about the outcome of routine activities, in particular those associated with the health of or separation from loved ones. Some people often anticipate a catastrophic outcome from a mild physical symptom or a side effect of medication. Demoralization is said to be a common consequence, with many individuals becoming discouraged, ashamed and unhappy about the difficulties of carrying out their normal routines. GAD is often comorbid with depression, and this can make accurate diagnosis problematic (Wittchen et al. 2002).

Exclusion criteria: The symptoms are not a manifestation of another health condition and are not due to the effects of a substance or medication on the central nervous system. In addition, ruling out the characteristics of other mental health diagnoses is important – e.g. disorders where anxiety and worry is also present, for example panic disorder associated with having panic attacks or social anxiety typified by being embarrassed in social situations.

Panic disorder

Panic disorder is characterized by recurrent unexpected panic attacks that are not restricted to particular stimuli or situations. Panic attacks are discrete episodes of intense fear or apprehension accompanied by the rapid and concurrent onset of several characteristic symptoms, e.g. palpitations or increased heart rate, sweating, trembling, shortness of breath, chest pain, dizziness or lightheadedness, chills, hot flushes, fear of imminent death. In addition, panic disorder is characterized by persistent concern about the recurrence or significance of panic attacks, or behaviours intended to avoid their recurrence. Note that triggers can be situational or external, including a feared object or particular situation, or internal, including catastrophic misinterpretation of physiological symptoms. This can lead to avoidance of situations in an attempt to prevent the panic attacks reoccurring, although this is largely ineffective as the individual may still experience panic (Breier et al. 1986). As with all anxiety disorders, this can lead to significant impairment in family, social, educational, workplace or other areas of functioning.

Exclusion criteria: The symptoms are not a manifestation of another medical condition or a result of a substance or medication affecting the central nervous system. These symptoms are not those that indicate a heart attack – although the symptoms of a heart attack and panic attack are similar, there are marked differences including the intensity of pain in the chest region worsen in a heart attack, and the symptoms are not short-lived (Carleton et al. 2014).

Obsessive-compulsive disorder

Obsessive-compulsive disorder (OCD) is characterized by the presence of obsessions, compulsions or both.

An obsession can be defined as an unwanted intrusive thought, image or urge that regularly goes through the individual's mind, rather than originating from an external source. Obsessions can be highly distressing and are considered as being unreasonable or excessive. Examples of obsessions include, but are not limited to, contamination from dirt, fear of harm, excessive focus on order or orderliness, obsessions with the body, intrusive thoughts (e.g. of committing a crime or hurting someone or something) (Lochner and Stein 2003).

Compulsions are repetitive behaviours or mental acts that an individual feels they have to perform. A compulsion can either be overt and observable by others, or a covert mental compulsion that cannot be observed. Common compulsions include checking, cleaning, washing, or mental compulsions such as counting, ordering, symmetry or exactness, hoarding (Foa et al. 1995). Some of these symptoms are missed or dismissed as normal behaviour.

Exclusion criteria: A compulsion is not in itself pleasurable, which differentiates it from impulsive acts such as shopping or gambling, which are associated with immediate gratification.

Post-traumatic stress disorder

Post-traumatic stress disorder (PTSD) often develops following exposure to an extremely threatening – e.g. life-threatening or horrific – event or series of events (Foa et al. 2008). This may include, but is not exclusive to, those exposed to violent crime, refugees, armed forces personnel, traumatic childbirth, or emergency service personnel. As noted in ICD-11, it is characterized by all of the following:

1 re-experiencing the traumatic event or events in the present in the form of vivid intrusive memories, flashbacks, or nightmares. Re-experiencing may occur via one or multiple sensory modalities and is typically accompanied by strong or overwhelming emotions, particularly fear or horror, and strong physical sensations;
2 avoidance of thoughts and memories of the event or events, or avoidance of activities, situations, or people reminiscent of the event(s); and
3 persistent perceptions of heightened current threat, for example as indicated by hypervigilance or an enhanced startle reaction to stimuli such as unexpected noises. The symptoms persist for at least several weeks and cause significant impairment in personal, family, social, educational, occupational or other important areas of functioning. (WHO 2018)

As a consequence, the individual may become hypervigilant to threats, experience inflated startle responses, irritability, difficulty in concentrating, sleep problems and avoid reminders of the trauma. It is commonplace for individuals with PTSD to report feeling emotionally numb, including an inability to feel, feelings of detachment from others around them and amnesia in some cases. As a result, low mood or depression symptoms can also occur, especially if the individual stops engaging in activities they once took part in.

Exclusion criteria: The symptoms are not those specific to acute stress reaction or complex post-traumatic stress disorder.

Social anxiety disorder

Social anxiety disorder is characterized by marked and excessive fear or anxiety that invariably occurs in one or more social situations. This includes social interactions, taking part in an activity where one feels observed or performing in front of others. The individual is preoccupied that they will be judged negatively if they display anxiety symptoms, and feeling embarrassed or humiliated is commonplace. This can be triggered by the actual or imagined scrutiny from others. As a result, the individual may avoid social situations, or if they cannot avoid them they will experience fear or anxiety. These symptoms usually persist for several months and can lead to significant impairment in family, social, educational, workplace, or other areas of functioning. Social anxiety disorder is characterized by a range of physical symptoms including excessive blushing, sweating, trembling, palpitations and nausea.

Exclusion criteria: Ruling out other mental health problems may be helpful as well as acknowledging comorbidities. This may include panic attacks and depressive symptoms as these difficulties may develop consequently. The individual may also misuse alcohol or drugs to cope with the difficulties.

Mood disorders

Mood disorders are typified by a loss of interest, pleasure and enjoyment in activities the individual usually undertakes. This can include: difficulty in concentrating, changes in appetite, poor sleep (e.g. sleeping too much or too little), a sense of worthlessness, thoughts of wanting to hurt themselves or end their life.

Mood disorders are subdivided into the following:

- major depressive episodes
- manic episodes
- mixed episodes
- hypomanic episodes

As you read the case study consider the risk and protective factors.

Case study 4.2 Depression

Karl (45 years old) has increasingly become withdrawn from friends and family – even his work colleagues have noticed that he's distant. He has been increasingly expressing a sense of hopelessness about the future. Around five years ago he lost his 5 year old son to leukaemia and his marriage of two years broke down shortly afterwards. At this time, he withdrew from everything and everyone until his parents encouraged him to seek support. Karl visited his GP, who prescribed an antidepressant and encouraged him to also attend one-to-one therapy via a local charity. He subsequently began a new routine that included progressing his accountancy career, taking up cycling with a local group, and a year ago started dating Sally. Two months ago Karl developed seasonal flu symptoms and took a week off work. During this time he stopped taking his antidepressant, began losing interest in his day-to-day life and started withdrawing from people around him. The company he worked for made him redundant and he has been arguing with his girlfriend. One Saturday night around the anniversary of the death of his son, he connected a hose from the exhaust pipe into the window of his car and switched on the engine in his garage. His neighbour saw smoke from the garage and rang an ambulance. Karl was found semi-conscious.

Points to consider: Being mindful of undermining the severity of the individual's situation and also overly identifying with their situation.

Depression

Depression is typified by the absence of positive affect, the loss of interest and enjoyment in everyday experiences, low mood and a range of associated emotional, cognitive, physical and behavioural symptoms. For these to be clinically significant the symptoms would usually exist over a significant period of time and have a severe impact (Lewinsohn et al. 2000). During a major depressive episode the individual is typically unreactive to their situation and will remain low in mood throughout the day (although note that this may be characterized by consistent low mood or a slight improvement with returning low mood the following day). An improvement in mood is usually not sustained and low mood returns within a short period (Andrews and Jenkins 1999). Table 4.3 summarizes the associated emotional, cognitive, physical and behavioural symptoms (Gerber et al. 1992; Cassano and Fava 2002). A lack of libido, fatigue and diminished activity are also common, although agitation and marked anxiety can frequently occur. Typically there is reduced sleep and lowered appetite (sometimes leading to significant weight loss), but some people sleep more than usual and have an increase in appetite. A loss of interest and enjoyment in everyday life, and feelings of guilt, worthlessness and deserved punishment are common, as are lowered self-esteem, loss of confidence, feelings of helplessness, suicidal ideation and attempts at self-harm or suicide. Cognitive changes include poor concentration and reduced attention, pessimistic and recurrently negative thoughts about oneself, one's past and the future, mental slowing and rumination (Cassano and Fava 2002).

Table 4.3 A summary of emotional, cognitive, physical and **behavioural symptoms**

Behavioural	Physical	Cognitive	Emotional
Tearfulness, irritability, poor appetite, withdrawn and loss of interest in activities, poor sleep	Increased muscle tension, pre-existing or new muscular pains, fatigue, weight loss	Reduced concentration and attention, poor memory, negative thought patterns	Hopelessness, worthlessness, anger, guilt, anxiety, low self-esteem

Gerber et al. 1992; Cassano and Fava 2002

As part of assessing a patient a paramedic could ask the following broad questions (adapted from Spitzer et al. 1994).

A line of questioning for depression:

- Has anything happened to trigger you feeling this way?
- During the last month, have you often been bothered by feeling down, depressed or hopeless?
- During the last month, have you often been bothered by having little interest or pleasure in doing things?

A line of questioning for anxiety:

- Has anything happened to trigger you feeling this way?
- Have you been feeling nervous, anxious or on edge?
- Have you been feeling afraid as if something terrible will happen?

NB: With the patient's consent, this may include asking family, carers and friends.

Severe and enduring mental health problems

By definition, severe mental illness (SMI) is recognized as non-organic in origin, meaning that it is not a result of brain disease such as dementia. In addition, it is characterized as being long-standing, of at least two years in duration, and meets the criteria as outlined in DSM-V or ICD-11.

Rehabilitation for people with severe and enduring mental illness is usually provided in a care pathway that includes inpatient and community-based rehabilitation services.

Although this book is an introduction, it is important to understand what severe and enduring mental health conditions are and how they differ from common mental health conditions. Given the significant impairment due to this category of mental health difficulties, consideration may need to be given to whether the person has capacity (please see Chapter 2). Similar to common mental health problems, there are different subtypes of SMI which we will explore under each diagnosis. As a starting point, Table 4.4 provides an overall summary of the most frequently referred to severe and enduring mental health problems.

Table 4.4 A summary of severe and enduring mental health problems

Schizophrenia	Personality disorders
Psychosis	Bipolar disorder
Dual diagnosis	Eating disorders

As part of assessing a patient, a paramedic could ask the following broad questions:

- Have you experienced these symptoms before?
- Do you know what might have triggered your symptoms on this occasion?

Schizophrenia

Diagnosis and characteristics

Schizophrenia is associated with other primary psychotic disorders, which are characterized by significant impairment to experience of reality and altered behaviour. These are generally organized into positive and negative symptoms such as those listed in Table 4.5, where it is recognized that the intensity and frequency of such symptoms deviate sufficiently from the expected cultural or subcultural norms.

Table 4.5 Positive and negative symptoms associated with schizophrenia

Positive symptoms	Negative symptoms
Persistent delusions, persistent hallucinations, disorganized thinking (typically manifest as disorganized speech), grossly disorganized behaviour, and experiences of passivity and control	Blunted or flat affect and avolition, and psychomotor disturbances

Adapted from WHO (2018); Katona et al. (2015)

Exclusion criteria: These symptoms should not result from features of another mental or behavioural disorder, such as but not limited to mood disorder, delirium, or a disorder due to substance use. ICD-11 also states that the categories in this grouping should not be used to classify the expression of ideas, beliefs or behaviours that are culturally sanctioned (WHO 2018).

Aetiology

Genetics: The prevalence of schizophrenia and other primary psychotic disorders increases for individuals who have a family history of the diagnosis.

As you read the case study, consider what your role might be when you receive the call and then arrive on scene.

Case study 4.3 Schizophrenia

John (51 years old) was diagnosed with schizophrenia when he was 25. John had a stable upbringing, raised on a working farm, and was an only child. He attended school achieving good grades, although his reports would often state that John was a daydreamer and not engaged with his peer group. John left as soon as he could to work with his dad on the farm. His mum was unwell for long periods throughout his childhood, staying with her family who live many miles away to recuperate. Although his mum was loving towards John, she was often vacant and distant when she was home. John didn't mind because he was very close to his dad. John's mum died by suicide just before his 23rd birthday. As John got older his dad would be away from home to buy and sell livestock, trusting John to look after the farm, although he had staff to help him. On various occasions the farm staff reported that John was displaying unusual behaviour, talking to people that weren't there and appearing to follow their instructions. This also meant that the farm staff were having to do John's work as well as their own. They also described finding him dressed only in his underwear when the temperatures dropped to below freezing, and times when he appeared to be up at all hours. John's dad dismissed it at first; however, on witnessing increasing risk-taking behaviours, including John taking steps to end his life, he urgently contacted John's GP who referred him to the crisis team. Subsequently John undertook various assessments over a period of months and a psychiatrist recognized the symptoms over his life course as schizophrenia. John received appropriate care that meant he could continue to live at home and his dad became his main carer. John's dad has just turned 80 years old and is struggling to care for himself and John, despite having carers visit daily. John's dad recently needed to have an operation and a short hospital stay, and during this time John forgot to take his medication even though his carers reminded him. John's symptoms worsened and his neighbours called for the emergency services after they witnessed him displaying unusual behaviour and threatening them with a spade. John was taken to a place of safety and assessed.

Pause for reflection

What might be some of the risk factors John presents with? What might be some of the protective factors John highlights?

Psychosis

Diagnosis and characteristics

ICD-11 refers to psychosis as acute and transient psychotic disorder (WHO 2018). It is characterized by acute onset of psychotic symptoms that emerge without any early symptoms indicating onset – what's known as a prodrome. The severity of the symptoms peaks within two weeks. Symptoms include hallucinations, delusions, disorganized patterns of thinking, confusion or incomprehension, and catatonia may also be present. Note that the intensity of symptoms is changeable, often within a short time frame. The duration of a psychotic episode is typically up to a month, and not exceeding three months.

Research has shown there is often a considerable time between the first presentation of symptoms and subsequent diagnosis of a first episode of psychosis – e.g. one year. This can lead to a delay in treatment and worsen outcomes (Souaiby et al. 2016; Chen et al. 2019).

Exclusion criteria: These symptoms should not be a manifestation of another medical condition and are not a result of a substance or medication affecting the central nervous system, including withdrawal.

Personality disorders

Diagnosis and characteristics

Personality disorder is characterized by problems in the functioning of all aspects of 'self' and interpersonal dysfunction. It is anticipated that these difficulties would have occurred over two years or more. This includes but is not limited to the symptoms outlined in Table 4.6.

Table 4.6 Symptoms that characterize personality disorders

Aspects of self	Interpersonal dysfunction
Self-identity	Ability to develop and maintain close and mutually
Self-worth	fulfilling relationships
Self-direction	Poor management of conflict in relationships
Accuracy of self-view	A reduced ability to understand others' perspectives

Adapted from WHO (2018)

The problems are likely to appear in patterns of cognition, emotional experience and expression, and maladaptive behaviour, across different social and personal situations. These are likely to be noted as inflexible and dysregulated. The problems are usually associated with significant distress or impairment in an important area of functioning, e.g. occupation or education setting, family.

Exclusion criteria: The patterns of behaviour characterizing the disturbance are not developmentally appropriate and cannot be explained primarily by social or cultural factors, including sociopolitical conflict.

ICD-11 notes the diagnosis as mild, moderate and severe, where the general diagnostic criteria are met with variations in intensity, as Table 4.7 outlines.

Table 4.7 Criteria that characterize mild, moderate and severe personality disorders

Mild personality disorder	Moderate personality disorder	Severe personality disorder
Problems are limited to some areas of functioning and thus may not be evident in some situations	Problems appear in multiple areas of functioning, however some areas of functioning are less affected	There are severe disturbances in functioning of the self and interpersonal functioning
Problems may occur in one or more areas, however functioning is maintained	Relationships and performance are likely to be characterized by disruption	There is severe impairment in nearly all areas of life

(Continued)

Table 4.7   (Continued)

Mild personality disorder	Moderate personality disorder	Severe personality disorder
Substantial harm to self or others is largely absent, but may be triggered by significant distress	On occasion this is associated with harm to self or others	There is often association with harm to self or others

Adapted from WHO (2018)

Bipolar disorder

Diagnosis and characteristics

Bipolar disorders are recognized as episodic mood disorders, characterized by the occurrence of manic, mixed or hypomanic episodes or symptoms. Such episodes typically alternate over the course of these disorders with episodes or periods of depressive symptoms. ICD-11 separates the diagnosis into type I and type II, as explored below.

Bipolar type I disorder

A type I bipolar disorder is characterized by the occurrence of one or more manic or mixed episodes – a diagnosis can be made based on evidence of a single manic or mixed episode. More typically, though, this diagnosis occurs with manic or mixed episodes cycling with depressive episodes over the course of the disorder (WHO 2018).

Table 4.8   Characteristics of bipolar type I disorder

A manic episode	A mixed episode
Characterized by euphoria, irritability or expansiveness, and by increased activity or a subjective experience of increased energy, accompanied by other characteristic symptoms such as rapid or pressured speech, flight of ideas, increased self-esteem or grandiosity, decreased need for sleep, distractibility, impulsive or reckless behaviour, and rapid changes among different mood states (i.e. mood lability).	Characterized by either a mixture of or very rapid cycling between prominent manic and depressive symptoms.
Duration: continues for at least one week.	**Duration:** occurs on most days during a period of at least two weeks.

Adapted from WHO (2018)

Bipolar type II disorder

Type II bipolar disorders are characterized by the occurrence of one or more hypomanic episodes and at least one depressive episode.

Table 4.9   Characteristics of bipolar type II disorder

A hypomanic episode	A depressive episode
A hypomanic episode is a persistent mood state characterized by persistent elevation of mood or increased irritability as well as increased activity or a subjective experience of increased energy. This often includes other characteristic symptoms such as an increase in talking, racing thoughts, increased self-esteem, a reduction in the need for sleep, being easily distracted and impulsive behaviour.	A depressive episode is characterized by a period of daily or almost daily depressed mood. This includes reduced interest in daily activities and occurs with other symptoms including poor appetite or sleep, agitation or slowing of psychomotor function, fatigue, excessive feelings of worthlessness or inappropriate feelings of guilt, hopelessness, poor concentration and suicidal ideation.
Duration: symptoms last for at least several days.	**Duration:** symptoms are almost daily and last for at least two weeks.

Adapted from WHO (2018)

Exclusion criteria: There is no history of manic or mixed episodes, and although the symptoms differ from the individual's typical mood, energy and behaviour, they are not severe enough to cause marked impairment in functioning.

Feeding and eating disorders

Diagnosis and characteristics

Feeding and eating disorders are both associated with abnormal feeding or eating behaviours, however ICD-11 differentiates between the two (WHO 2018). Feeding disorders are identified as behavioural difficulties including, but not limited to, eating non-edible substances or voluntary regurgitation of foods, that is unrelated to body weight and shape concerns. Eating disorders involve abnormal eating behaviour and preoccupation with food as well as prominent body weight and shape concerns (WHO 2018). There are a number of different eating disorders, however the authors would like to focus on two that are most frequently in contact with pre-hospital care, anorexia nervosa and bulimia nervosa.

Anorexia nervosa is characterized by significantly low body weight (most frequently measured by body mass index (BMI)) – in adults a BMI of less than 18.5 kg/m^2 and in children and young people BMI-for-age under 5th percentile. Low body weight is accompanied by a persistent pattern of behaviours to prevent normal weight gain or maintenance of a healthy weight. This may include behaviours aimed at restricted eating, purging behaviours and behaviours such as excessive exercise. These behaviours are typically associated with a fear of weight gain. Low body weight or body shape is central to the person's self-judgement or is inaccurately perceived to be normal or even overweight.

Rapid weight loss, such as more than 20 per cent of total body weight within six months, may replace the low body weight guideline in addition to other diagnostic requirements. But it is important to note that, specific to children and young people, they may fail to gain weight as expected based on their individual developmental trajectory, rather than due to weight loss.

Pre-hospital care requirements: An individual with anorexia nervosa may be experiencing major organ failure. Monitoring physical signs and using a central venous line may be difficult due to low blood pressure.

Bulimia nervosa is characterized by frequent, recurrent episodes of binge eating. Usually this occurs at least once a week over a period of at least one month. A binge eating episode is typified by a perceived loss of control over eating, such as eating notably more or differently and feeling unable to stop or limit the type of food eaten. Binge eating is accompanied by compensatory behaviours to prevent weight gain. This may include self-induced vomiting, misuse of laxatives or enemas, and strenuous exercise. The individual is fixated on their weight and/or body shape and this drives negative self-evaluation. The individual may experience significant distress about their behaviours, including embarrassment and guilt. There is often significant impairment in wider areas of life including relationships and occupation.

In order to gain a diagnosis of bulimia nervosa the individual should not meet the diagnostic requirements of anorexia nervosa.

Pre-hospital care requirements: An individual with bulimia nervosa may have a tear in their oesophagus or bleeding from the stomach lining.

Exclusion criteria: Symptoms that are not explained by another health condition and are not developmentally appropriate or culturally sanctioned or due to the unavailability of food.

Substance use

Disorders due to substance use are characterized by single episodes of harmful substance use, or substance use disorders, which encompass harmful substance use and substance dependence. They can also include substance-induced disorders such as substance intoxication, substance withdrawal and substance-induced mental disorders, sexual dysfunction and sleep–wake disorders. Diagnostic criteria identify several categories associated with different types of substance use, however the authors have focused on alcohol and stimulants as examples (WHO 2018).

Alcohol dependence

Alcohol dependence is a disorder associated with regulation of alcohol use arising from either continuous or repeated alcohol use. There is a strong internal drive to use alcohol, which is maintained by an inability to control that use despite the harm caused – the individual's focus is on alcohol, often at the expense of other functioning. There may be the presence craving alcohol present in physiological features of dependence, including tolerance or withdrawal symptoms. This usually occurs over a period of at least 12 months but can also happen if alcohol use is continuous for at least one month.

Korsakoff syndrome is a disease of the nervous system, caused by deficiency of vitamin B1, and may be characterized by an inability to form new memories, amnesia, confabulation or hallucinations. Chronic alcohol use may be associated with thiamine deficiency, but alcohol may also have effects on the brain via other mechanisms.

Harmful pattern of use of stimulants including amphetamines, methamphetamine or methcathinone

The use of stimulants including amphetamines, methamphetamine and methcathinone may have caused damage to a individual's physical or mental health over a period of at least one year. This may have also resulted in behaviour leading to harm to others. Risk to health may occur due to:

1. behaviour related to intoxication;
2. direct or secondary toxic effects on body organs and systems; or
3. a harmful route of administration. Harm to health of others includes any form of physical harm, including trauma, or mental disorder that is directly attributable to behaviour related to stimulant intoxication on the part of the person to whom the diagnosis of Harmful pattern of use of stimulants including amphetamines, methamphetamine and methcathinone applies. (WHO 2018)

Beyond mental health: the interaction between mental health and physical health

While this book is focused on mental health, the authors recognize that the interaction between mental health and physical health is an important one to mention. Misdiagnosis can occur or a diagnosis can be misunderstood, which can lead to unintended consequences such as delay in recovery, unnecessary admission to hospital or readmissions. Therefore, the following section will briefly explore dementia and developmental disorders.

Dementia

Dementia is recognized as a progressive and irreversible condition, characterized by a deterioration in cognitive, behavioural and psychological functioning, as well as a loss of identity, including independence. Individuals with dementia are more likely to have chronic disease and therefore experience more health difficulties that may in turn impact on their mental health (Sanderson et al. 2002; Schubert et al. 2006; Zhao et al. 2008; Poblador-Plou et al. 2014). It is known that individuals with comorbidities that include dementia are more likely to access emergency services (Phelan et al. 2012; Voss et al. 2017). Therefore, pre-hospital care is an important consideration with this diagnosis (Zhao et al. 2008; Phelan et al. 2012; Wittenberg et al. 2019).

Research has shown that the 'conversion rate', or the proportion of A&E attendances arriving by ambulance that become hospital admissions, is high in this patient group (Wittenberg et al. 2019). In addition, readmission rates for this diagnosis are high. Some of these admissions could be seen as unnecessary. Transport to hospital in an ambulance can be particularly distressing and lead to behavioural disturbances (Ferns 2006; Hodge and Marshall 2007; Gitlin et al. 2008). Dementia can provide many challenges to pre-hospital care, such as difficulties gaining a medical history. It is also possible that the diagnosis of dementia can act to mask other symptoms – what is sometimes termed 'diagnostic overshadowing' (Jones et al. 2008; Van Nieuwenhuizen et al. 2013). These factors could lead to adverse clinical outcomes and readmission. Therefore, to improve outcomes and experiences for patients and carers, reducing hospital admission is favourable.

Neurodevelopmental disorders

ICD-11 recognizes neurodevelopmental disorders as behavioural and cognitive disorders that occur during the developmental period and involve significant difficulties in the development of specific intellectual, motor, language or social functions. There are different types of neurodevelopmental disorders, however the following will focus on learning disabilities.

Learning disabilities

A learning disability is recognized as a type of neurodevelopmental disorder. There is evidence to suggest that common mental health disorders, including cognitive and behavioural difficulties, are present in adults with learning disabilities (Cooper et al. 2007). The prevalence and severity of these difficulties is often dependent on the severity of the learning disabilities (Whitaker and Read 2006). However, given the nature of the learning disability the accuracy of the assessment and diagnosis is questionable (Smiley 2005; Whitaker and Read 2006). This can present different challenges in pre-hospital care, such as accuracy of medical diagnosis. As mentioned above, 'diagnostic overshadowing' must be a consideration when assessing the individual.

Exclusion criteria: Note that many people with mental and behavioural disorders also have behavioural and cognitive deficits present during the developmental period. However, only disorders whose core features are neurodevelopmental are included.

Aetiology: This is complex and in many individual cases is unknown.

The contested position of diagnostic criteria

While there are many functional aspects of having diagnostic criteria in place, it is important to consider other perspectives when evaluating effective care. There is much criticism of the development, application and future of diagnostic criteria. This alone highlights the great significance diagnostic criteria have in society. For example, if an individual's narrative is excluded this could be viewed as restrictive practice. Similarly, from a sociological perspective diagnosis is stipulated as a control or oppressive mechanism. The role of the media in its portrayal of mental health diagnoses also contributes to popularist schools of thought. For example, a popular television series that emphasizes the link between criminality and schizophrenia arguably forms a negative construct. Therefore, the contested nature of diagnosis within mental health can be seen from the perspectives of biological, psychological and social schools of thought.

In conclusion: the future of diagnostic criteria

This chapter has outlined the operational components of diagnostic criteria, while emphasizing the importance of other perspectives, in the provision of effective care. In offering alternative perspectives it is evident that there are contrasting positions and thus criticisms of using diagnostic criteria. While a diagnostic-centred approach might forget to take a holistic or whole person approach, taking a whole person approach might miss important details and be critiqued as reductionist. Through taking different perspectives in the diagnosis of mental health conditions, we may in turn challenge the way we see diagnosis and continue to develop patient-centred recovery.

The chapter has highlighted overlap between some medical diagnoses and different mental health difficulties. This can lead to misdiagnosis and delay in treatment plans, and on occasion some diagnoses take many years to be formalized, as other conditions need to be ruled out. The impact on the individual, family and friends is significant and can include a change of role and responsibilities. For example, an individual may become a full-time carer if the needs of the individual increase. Therefore, consideration needs to be given to the roles of those involved in pre-hospital care where possible.

References

Andrews, G. and Jenkins, R. (eds) (1999) *Management of Mental Disorders*, 1st edn. Sydney: WHO Collaborating Centre for Mental Health and Substance Misuse/Geneva: World Health Organization.

Augustus, J., Bold, J. and Williams, B. (2019) *An Introduction to Mental Health*. London: Sage.

Banwell, E., Humphrey, N. and Qualter, P. (2021) Delivering and implementing child and adolescent mental health training for mental health and allied professionals: A systematic review and qualitative meta-aggregation, *BMC Medical Education*, 21(1): 103.

Biederman, J., Monuteaux, M.C., Spencer, T. et al. (2009) Do stimulants protect against psychiatric disorders in youth with ADHD? A 10-year follow-up study, *Pediatrics*, 124(1): 71–8.

Breier, A., Charney, D.S. and Heninger, G.R. (1986) Agoraphobia with panic attacks: Development, diagnostic stability, and course of illness, *Archives of General Psychiatry*, 43(11): 1029–36.

Brown, T.A., O'Leary, T.A. and Barlow, D.H. (2001) Generalised anxiety disorder, in D.H. Barlow (ed.) *Clinical Handbook of Psychological Disorders: A Step-by-Step Treatment Manual*, 3rd edn. New York: Guilford Press, pp. 154–208.

Carleton, R.N., Duranceau, S., Freeston, M.H., Boelen, P.A., McCabe, R.E. and Antony, M.M. (2014) "But it might be a heart attack": Intolerance of uncertainty and panic disorder symptoms, *Journal of Anxiety Disorders*, 28(5): 463-70.

Cassano, P. and Fava, M. (2002) Depression and public health: An overview, *Journal of Psychosomatic Research*, 53(4): 849–57.

Chen, Y., Farooq, S., Edwards, J. et al. (2019) Patterns of symptoms before a diagnosis of first episode psychosis: A latent class analysis of UK primary care electronic health records, *BMC Medicine*, 17(1): 227.

Cohen, D.A., Klodnick, V.V., Kramer, M.D., Strakowski, S.M. and Baker, J. (2020) Predicting child-to-adult community mental health service continuation, *Journal of Behavioral Health Services & Research*, 47(3): 331–45.

Cooper, S.-A., Smiley, E., Morrison, J., Williamson, A. and Allan, L. (2007) Mental ill-health in adults with intellectual disabilities: Prevalence and associated factors, *British Journal of Psychiatry*, 190(1): 27–35.

Duffy, A. (2012) The nature of the association between childhood ADHD and the development of bipolar disorder: A review of prospective high-risk studies, *American Journal of Psychiatry*, 169(12): 1247–55.

Duffy, A., Horrocks, J., Doucette, S., Keown-Stoneman, C, McCloskey, S. and Grof, P. (2014) The developmental trajectory of bipolar disorder, *British Journal of Psychiatry*, 204(2): 122–8.

Duong, M.T., Bruns, E.J., Lee, K. et al. (2021) Rates of mental health service utilization by children and adolescents in schools and other common service settings: A systematic review and meta-analysis, *Administration and Policy in Mental Health Services Research*, 48(3): 420–39.

Ferns, T. (2006) Violence, aggression and physical assault in healthcare settings, *Nursing Standard*, 21(13): 42–6.

Foa, E.B., Keane, T.M. and Friedman, M.J. (2008) *Effective Treatments for PTSD: Practice Guidelines from the International Society for Traumatic Stress Studies*. New York: Guilford Press.

Foa, E.B., Kozak, M.J., Goodman, W.K., Hollander, E., Jenike, M.A. and Rasmussen, S.A. (1995) DSM-IV field trial: Obsessive compulsive disorder, *American Journal of Psychiatry*, 152(1): 90–6.

Gerber, P.D., Barrett, J.E., Barrett, J.A., et al. (1992) The relationship of presenting physical complaints to depressive symptoms in primary care patients, *Journal of General Internal Medicine*, 7(2): 170–3.

Gitlin, L.N., Winter, L., Burke, J., Chernett, N., Dennis, M.P. and Hauck, W. (2008) Tailored activities to manage neuropsychiatric behaviors in persons with dementia and reduce caregiver burden: A randomized pilot study, *American Journal of Geriatric Psychiatry*, 16(3): 229–39.

Hodge, A.N. and Marshall, A.P. (2007) Violence and aggression in the emergency department: A critical care perspective, *Aust Crit Care*, 20(2): 61–7.

Jones, S., Howard, L. and Thornicroft, G. (2008) 'Diagnostic overshadowing': Worse physical health care for people with mental illness, *Acta Psychiatr Scand*, 118(3): 169–71.

Katona, C.L.E., Cooper, C. and Robertson, M.M. (2015) *Psychiatry at a Glance*, 6th edn. Chichester: Wiley Blackwell.

Kendrick, T. and Pilling, S. (2012) Common mental health disorders — identification and pathways to care: NICE clinical guideline, *British Journal of General Practice*, 62(594): 47–9.

Kessler, R.C., Angermeyer, M., Anthony, J.C. et al. (2007) Lifetime prevalence and age-of-onset distributions of mental disorders in the World Health Organization's World Mental Health Survey Initiative, *World Psychiatry*, 6(3): 168–76.

Lewinsohn, P.M., Solomon, A., Seeley, J.R. and Zeiss, A. (2000) Clinical implications of 'subthreshold' depressive symptoms, *Journal of Abnormal Psychology*, 109(2): 345–51.

Lochner, C. and Stein, D.J. (2003) Heterogeneity of obsessive-compulsive disorder: A literature review, *Harvard Review of Psychiatry*, 11(3): 113–32.

National Institute for Health and Care Excellence (NICE) (2011) *Common Mental Health Disorders: Identification and Pathways to Care*. Clinical guideline CG123. London: NICE. Available at: http://guidance.nice.org.uk/CG123 (accessed 3 September 2020).

Phelan, E.A., Borson, S., Grothaus, L., Balch, S. and Larson, E.B. (2012) Association of incident dementia with hospitalizations, *JAMA*, 307(2): 165–72.

Poblador-Plou, B., Calderón-Larrañaga, A., Marta-Moreno, J. et al. (2014) Comorbidity of dementia: A cross-sectional study of primary care older patients, *BMC Psychiatry*, 14(1): 84.

Rolfe, U., Pope, C. and Crouch, R. (2020) Paramedic performance when managing patients experiencing mental health issues – exploring paramedics' presentation of self, *International Emergency Nursing*, 49: 100828.

Sanderson, M., Wang, J., Davis, D.R., Lane, M.J., Cornman, C.B. and Fadden, M.K. (2002) Co-morbidity associated with dementia, *American Journal of Alzheimer's Disease and other Dementias*, 17(2): 73–8.

Schubert, C.C., Boustani, M., Callahan, C.M. et al. (2006) Comorbidity profile of dementia patients in primary care: Are they sicker?, *Journal of the American Geriatrics Society*, 54(1): 104–9.

Smiley, E. (2005) Epidemiology of mental health problems in adults with learning disabilities: An update, *Advances in Psychiatric Treatment*, 11(3): 214–22.

Souaiby, L., Gaillard, R. and Krebs, M.O. (2016) Duration of untreated psychosis: A state-of-the-art review and critical analysis, *Encephale*, 42(4): 361–6.

Spitzer, R.L., Williams, J.B., Kroenke, K. et al. (1994) Utility of a new procedure for diagnosing mental disorders in primary care. The PRIME-MD 1000 study, *JAMA*, 272(22): 1749–56.

Van Nieuwenhuizen, A., Henderson, C., Kassam, A. et al. (2013) Emergency department staff views and experiences on diagnostic overshadowing related to people with mental illness, *Epidemiology and Psychiatric Sciences*, 22(3): 255–62.

Voss, S., Black, S., Brandling, J. et al. (2017) Home or hospital for people with dementia and one or more other multimorbidities: What is the potential to reduce avoidable emergency admissions? The HOMEWARD Project Protocol, *BMJ Open*, 7(4): E016651.

Wadsworth, M.E. (2015) Development of maladaptive coping: A functional adaptation to chronic, uncontrollable stress, *Child Development Perspectives*, 9(2): 96–100. Available at: https://doi.org/10.1111/cdep.12112 (accessed 6 August 2021).

Waid, J. and Kelly, M. (2020) Supporting family engagement with child and adolescent mental health services: A scoping review, *Health & Social Care in the Community*, 28(5): 1333–42.

Whitaker, S. and Read, S. (2006) The prevalence of psychiatric disorders among people with intellectual disabilities: An analysis of the literature, *Journal of Applied Research in Intellectual Disabilities*, 19(4): 330–45.

Wittchen, H.U., Kessler, R.C., Beesdo, K., Krause, P., Höfler, M. and Hoyer, J. (2002) Generalised anxiety and depression in primary care: Prevalence, recognition, and management, *Journal of Clinical Psychiatry*, 63(Supp8): 24–34.

Wittenberg, R., Knapp, M., Hu, B. et al. (2019) The costs of dementia in England, *International Journal of Geriatric Psychiatry*, 34(7): 1095–103.

World Health Organization (WHO) (2018) *International Classification of Diseases for Mortality and Morbidity Statistics* (11th Revision). Available at: https://icd.who.int/browse11/l-m/en (accessed 31 October 2020).

World Health Organization (WHO) (2020) *Adolescent Mental Health*. Available at: https://www.who.int/news-room/fact-sheets/detail/adolescent-mental-health (accessed 23 June 2021).

Zhao, Y., Kuo, T.C., Weir, S., Kramer, M.S. and Ash, A.S. (2008) Healthcare costs and utilization for Medicare beneficiaries with Alzheimer's, *BMC Health Services Research*, 8: article 108.

5 Paramedic assessment

Paula Gardner

Learning objectives

- Explore the various assessment methods utilized by a range of healthcare professionals
- Look at the importance of the mental health assessment
- Highlight the methods which can be adapted to pre-hospital care
- Identify some of the skills that a paramedic can use when undertaking a mental health assessment
- Demonstrate how mental health assessment can contribute to the subsequent care of the patient
- Consider risk factors and challenges to the assessment process
- Explore the types of questions that can be used during the mental health assessment

Introduction

There are various methods of assessing mental health which are utilised in the private sector, primary care settings and the NHS. Assessments are conducted by practitioners such as psychologists, GPs, psychiatrists, mental health nurses and occupational therapists.

Ambulance clinicians can often be the first contact a patient suffering with a mental health condition has with health services, particularly with new or sudden onset of mental health disorders. Patients may display worrying behaviours which are concerning for those involved with the patient's care, such as relatives, carers or bystanders. There are many behavioural characteristics associated with mental health which could be related to other underlying causes. It is important to exclude medical or traumatic causes by conducting the relevant investigations and conveying the patient to an emergency department (ED) for further investigation if a medical or traumatic origin is suspected. Common behavioural characteristics for a variety of mental health conditions are reviewed in Chapter 4.

When attending to patients displaying mental health-related presentations, paramedic clinical practice is underpinned by clinical practice guidelines, organizational protocols and mental health legislation requirements (Shaban 2006). The management of mental health presentations is becoming an increasingly significant part of pre-hospital practice, but it is acknowledged that assessment and management of mental illness can be a challenge for paramedics (Lowthian et al. 2011).

Communication skills

How effectively psychological distress is assessed and subsequently managed is determined by the type of questions posed, the quality of the assessment and understanding what to look for in a patient. When carrying out the assessment of common mental health disorders, the clinician must be able to communicate effectively and possess the necessary skills required to perform an appropriate assessment (see Table 5.1).

Table 5.1 Skills required to perform an assessment

Points to consider	Skills to utilize
Risk assessment:	Verbal communication:
<ul><li>Is the patient safe? Consider the environment</li><li>Crew safety consideration – is egress clear?</li><li>Access to weapons available, including concealed weapons? (be cautious of hands/feet)</li><li>Patient's level of stress/anxiety</li><li>Is the patient angry?</li><li>Is the patient hallucinating? (can lead to violent or unpredictable behaviour)</li><li>Has the patient been using substances such as drugs or alcohol?</li><li>Is there a history of challenging or violent behaviour?</li></ul>	<ul><li>Be able to elicit the nature of the problem</li><li>Understand the patient's perception of the problem</li><li>Understand the impact of the condition on the patient</li><li>Avoid jargon</li><li>Use active listening skills</li><li>Minimal interruption – allow the patient to speak</li><li>Use silence appropriately</li><li>Put the patient at ease</li><li>Use questions that are easy to understand</li><li>Skills of negotiation with the patient or multi-professional team may be required</li></ul> Non-verbal communication: <ul><li>Face the patient and maintain eye contact where appropriate</li><li>Observe the patient and consider the environment</li></ul>

(Continued)

Points to consider	Skills to utilize
	• How does the patient appear – dressed appropriately?/unkempt?
	• Remain calm and non-judgemental
	• Open posture
	Other skills:
	• Ask the patient to sit and encourage them to remain calm
	• Adopt a warm approach
	• Offer reassurance
	• Be understanding
	• Take a holistic approach
	• Be sensitive to personal space
	• Undertake a mental capacity assessment
	• Are there any factors in the patient's environment causing them distress – relatives/bystanders present etc?

Patients will present in a variety of different ways and may be in significant distress, which can lead to difficulties in undertaking an assessment. It is important to successfully manage the distress and provide the highest standard of care (Trenoweth and Moone 2017).

In addition to assessing symptoms and associated functional impairment, the National Institute for Health and Care Excellence (NICE 2009) recommend that clinicians consider how the following factors may affect the development, course and severity of a person's presenting problem:

• A history of any mental health disorder
• A history of a chronic physical health problem
• Any past experience of, and responses to, treatments
• The quality of interpersonal relationships
• Living conditions and social isolation
• A family history of mental illness
• A history of domestic violence or sexual abuse
• Employment and immigration status

During the assessment process it is important to think about any children or young people who could be affected by the patient's condition and consider implementing local safeguarding procedures.

Psychosocial assessments in mental healthcare often involve the use of rating scales and assessment tools. NICE (2014) highlight that the aim of psychosocial assessments is to identify contributing factors which may explain issues such as self-harm and can also help patients begin the road to their recovery. There are a variety of mental health professionals who are trained in the assessment and treatment of mental health conditions. There are also different categories of mental health service provision:

- Primary care mental health – often through a GP
- Secondary care mental health – specialist services provided in the community or in hospital
- Community mental health team (CMHT) – a multidisciplinary team who work with adults with severe and enduring mental health problems

Mental health professionals

(See Chapter 2 for roles and responsibilities of different healthcare professionals.) In the pre-hospital environment, you may encounter some of the mental health workers involved in your patient's care, such as:

- Approved Mental Health Professional (AMHP)
- Psychiatrist
- Police officer
- Clinical and counselling psychologist
- Cognitive behaviour therapist
- Registered mental health nurse (RMN)
- Counsellor and psychotherapist
- Mental health social worker
- Occupational therapist (OT)
- Complementary and alternative medicine (CAM) practitioner

Mental capacity assessment

The Mental Capacity Act (MCA) (2005) in England and Wales sets out criteria for a test of capacity. This can be used as a guide for clinicians, enabling them to maintain a balance between promoting autonomy while also ensuring that care is provided in the 'best interests' of the patient, in the instance that they lack the capacity to make their own decisions.

The implementation of the MCA has resulted in a rise of interest in the concept of mental capacity, and its role in clinical decision-making and assessment in healthcare (Banner 2012). While people have the right to make what others might regard as an unwise decision, there are occasions when a person's refusal to consent to treatment will raise concerns about their ability to make a decision regarding their care. The assessment of capacity to consent to treatment is considered a fundamental component of shared practitioner patient deci-sion-making (Cliff and McGraw 2016). (See Chapter 2 for the principles of the MCA 2005).

The functional test of capacity

The purpose of the functional test of capacity is to:

- determine whether or not the person is able to make their own decision, and
- if they are not able to make their own decision, whether they are unable to do so as a result of the impairment or disturbance of their mind or brain

The functional test focuses on assessing a patient's ability using the following four factors:

1 The ability to understand information about the decision (the 'relevant' information)
2 The ability to retain the information long enough to make the decision
3 The ability to use, or 'weigh up' the information as part of the decision-making process
4 The ability to communicate their decision through any means

In order to make their own decision, the person must be able to demonstrate their ability in *all* of the areas of the functional test.

When carrying out the functional capacity test you have a duty to apply the first three statutory principles of the Act, as defined in Chapter 2.

It is important not to assess a person's understanding until they have been provided with all the relevant information to make the decision and all practi-cable steps have been taken to support them to understand it.

Case study 5.1

Howard is a 58 year old gentleman who has been experiencing several epi-sodes of central chest pain at rest. After conducting a set of observations, you advise Howard he needs to be taken to A&E for further investigations as you suspect he may be experiencing cardiac chest pain. Howard declines and states he would prefer to stay at home and continue to take paracetamol and Gaviscon. In order to assess whether Howard has the capacity to make this decision you need to apply the four elements of the functional test. How will you apply these to Howard? What questions will you ask Howard?

1 *The ability to understand information about the decision (the 'relevant' information)*
  Howard, if you do not attend A&E for further investigations you could have a myocardial infarction, which is a heart attack. This could mean that your

heart is damaged irreparably, or you could suffer a cardiac arrest. Can you explain back to me what might happen if you do not take the advice to attend hospital?

In order for a person to make their own decision they must be able to demonstrate all of the following:

- A general understanding of the decision to be made
- A general understanding about why the decision needs to be made
- A general understanding about the effects of deciding one way or the other, or of making no decision at all

2 *The ability to retain the information long enough to make the decision*
Wait for a few minutes and ask Howard to repeat back to you what might happen if he does not attend hospital.

In order to make their own decision the person needs to be able to demonstrate that they are able to retain (remember) the relevant information long enough to be able to make a decision. **There is no requirement for them to be able to retain the information longer than that.**

3 *The ability to use, or 'weigh up' the information as part of the decision-making process*
Is Howard able to make a decision on his treatment based on the information you have given him?

4 *The ability to communicate their decision through any means*
Can Howard communicate his decision back to you by using verbal or non-verbal communication methods?

According to the Mental Capacity Act (2005), very few people will be unable to communicate their decision *through any means*. The Code of Practice gives the following examples of where it would be appropriate to conclude that the person is unable to communicate their decision:

- When the person is unconscious or in a coma
- When the person is conscious but has a rare condition, such as 'locked in syndrome', that means they cannot speak or move at all

It is your responsibility to establish and take all practicable steps to:

- communicate with the person
- provide relevant information to the person
- support the person to communicate their decision

Everybody uses information differently when making a decision and it is important not to make a judgement about a person's ability to weigh up if they have not relayed the information in exactly the same way as you would have done (Mental Capacity Act 2005).

Mental health crisis

A definition of a mental health crisis is an acute disruption of psychological well-being in which usual coping mechanisms do not help the person overcome their feeling of distress (Yeager and Roberts 2015). Mental illness can be described as an alteration in a person's thinking, emotional regulation, or a behaviour, indicating an imbalance in their usual psychological functioning (Trenoweth and Moone 2017). This may include any of the conditions described in Chapter 4 such as generalized anxiety disorder and panic attacks, or psychotic episodes such as delusional thoughts, hallucinations, paranoia, hearing voices and mania. It may result in behaviour or acts such as suicide or self-harm. Mental health crisis is recognized as a psychiatric emergency requiring immediate specialist intervention (Wright and McGlen 2012).

Approaches to assessment

The assessment process can be complex and should be undertaken using a holistic, systematic approach (Trenoweth and Moone 2017). The process should begin with identifying the current issue and evaluating any risk to the person themselves or others. For the paramedic, the assessment and history taking will help to determine the most appropriate pathway for the patient (see Chapter 8 for further information on pathway referrals).

Approaches to assessment can be separated into three main categories: the comprehensive interview, observations and focused assessment tools. The comprehensive interview reviews all aspects of the person's bio-psycho-social functioning and is often used when a person is admitted as an inpatient to a mental health ward. The initial meeting will explore the patient's background and a health screen will be made. In addition, a doctor will carry out a detailed physical health assessment.

Observation of the patient's actions, manner, patterns of behaviour and speech might be used, for example, on an inpatient unit to regularly monitor the person's mood as part of the reassessment process. However, observation can also be used by the paramedic, to assess the person's mental state so that any improvement or deterioration can be identified while they are in their care.

The assessment will also review aspects of self-care such as: personal hygiene, nutrition, lifestyle, any changes to the person's pattern of living, socio-economic factors and any use of substances or alcohol. Organic causes should also be considered which can affect a patient's cognitive state, such as hypo/hyperglycaemia, hypoxia, common infections and neurological conditions, e.g. cerebral bleeding.

Assessment tools can be used that focus on a particular aspect of functioning. Assessment tools commonly consist of a number of specific questions and the responses are then tallied to reveal a total indicating the person's level of functioning at that point in time. This is the baseline score; often the same tool is later repeated to gauge if there has been any improvement or deterioration. There are a range of assessment tools used in healthcare settings to determine level of depression or risk of suicide. Let's take a look at some of the commonly used tools used to assess mental health to date.

The Global Mental Health Assessment Tool

In December 2016, the Home Office (HO) and Public Health England (PHE) in collaboration with the International Organization for Migration (IOM) began a pilot of the Global Mental Health Assessment Tool (GMHAT). The tool was used in the assessment of Syrian refugees who had claimed asylum in the United Kingdom. The GMHAT is a computerized clinical interview tool devised to rapidly identify a wide range of mental health problems in primary healthcare settings. The tool leads to a comprehensive but rapid mental state assessment. A report by the Home Office and PHE summarizes the findings of the evaluation around how this tool worked in practice at identifying immediate mental health needs that required urgent attention (HO, PHE and IOM 2017). The tool has been validated in primary care and specialist settings and across cultures.

The GMHAT consists of a series of questions focusing on the following symptoms or problems: worries, anxiety and panic attacks, concentration, depressed mood, sleep, appetite, eating disorders, hypochondriasis, obsessions and compulsions, phobias, mania/hypomania, thought disorders, psychotic symptoms, disorientation, memory impairment, alcohol and drug misuse, personality problems and stressors. The GMHAT produces a final assessment based on the person's responses, outlining any mental health problems, scoring against a range of mental health concerns, and an assessment of the severity of their symptoms.

According to Sharma et al. (2010), using an unstructured interview can lead to relevant information being missed from a patient's history. However, elements such as non-verbal cues can be missed when relying on computer-assisted questioning. They may also be perceived as an impersonal method of assessment.

The Patient Health Questionnaire (PHQ-9)

The PHQ-9 consists of nine questions and is used in primary care settings as a screening tool to measure the level of depression a patient has experienced over the last two weeks (Levis et al. 2019). The tool rates the frequency of symptoms of depression and assesses the presence of suicidal ideation. The PHQ-9 is completed by the patient and scored by the clinician. The patient indicates how often they have experienced the issues in each question, scoring 0 for not at all, 1 for several days, 2 for more than half the days and 3 for nearly every day:

1 Little interest or pleasure in doing things
2 Feeling down, depressed, or hopeless

3 Trouble falling or staying asleep, or sleeping too much

4 Feeling tired or having little energy

5 Poor appetite or overeating

6 Feeling bad about yourself or that you are a failure or have let yourself or your family down

7 Trouble concentrating on things, such as reading the newspaper or watching television

8 Moving or speaking so slowly that other people could have noticed, or the opposite: being so fidgety or restless that you have been moving around a lot more than usual

9 Thoughts that you would be better off dead, or of hurting yourself

The score is then interpreted using the following parameters:

1–4 = Minimal depression
5–9 = Mild depression
10–14 = Moderate depression
15–19 = Moderately severe depression
20–27 = Severe depression

Although the PHQ-9 tool is widely used and is a simple and quick method of assessing severity of depression, when Cameron et al. (2011) compared it with other commonly used assessment tools they found that the PHQ-9 often incorrectly categorized patients as experiencing a greater severity of symptoms. NICE (2009) state that the interpretation of assessment tools can be unreliable as a sole method of assessment, and factors such as functional impairment, history, family history and underlying medical conditions should also be considered.

Threshold Assessment Grid

The Threshold Assessment Grid (TAG) is used in general practice by a range of clinicians as a tool to assess the severity of a patient's mental health problems. The TAG score helps clinicians to ascertain suitability for psychological intervention by considering clinical findings, level of risk and patient safety (Jones and Greenberg 2015). The TAG comprises seven domains, each assessing safety, risk, needs and disabilities. Scores range from 0 to a maximum of 24. Findings can help with prioritization of treatment for those deemed at a higher clinical risk and need for interventions. Slade et al. (2000) believe the use of the TAG helps to reduce the issue of inappropriate referrals or mental health services receiving insufficient referral information.

Risk assessment matrix

The risk assessment matrix (RAM) was developed in 2004 at the Royal United Hospital for use in A&E departments as part of an initial assessment of mental health. The RAM assesses the patient's previous history and their appearance and behaviour, using a set of questions with free text space for the clinician's additional comments. The RAM is one of many tools that exist and is deemed a well-structured, easy-to-use adaptation which can be useful in assisting clinical decision-making (Patel et al. 2009).

Before some commonly used suicide risk assessment tools are reviewed, it is important to discuss self-harm and some of the considerations that should be taken into account as part of the assessment process.

Self-harm attempts

People who self-harm are often experiencing life problems such as relationship issues or other difficulties, and self-harm is often linked with suicide (Townsend et al. 2016). Self-harm is defined as the intentional act of self-injury (cutting, scratching, burning) or self-poisoning, carried out with or without suicidal intention (Harris et al. 2019). When attending suicide attempt cases, one priority for paramedics is to rapidly assess the level of physical risk the attempt may cause to the patient, as well as their current emotional state, providing transportation to A&E where appropriate. NICE (2004) recommends that most people who have taken overdoses or self-poisoned should be urgently taken to A&E due to the toxicity of the substance, which may be difficult to assess in the pre-hospital setting. If transportation to A&E is not deemed appropriate, paramedics should assess the patient for risk level and potential for re-attempting to harm themselves, psychosocial factors such as their personal situation and also establish the patient's access to a support network. It is important to convey this information to relevant services such as the patient's general practitioner (GP), out-of-hours GP, or other services such as crisis resolution teams. Consideration should be given to the toxic or potentially lethal dose of the ingested substance and the level of intent to end their life. Tools such as the IPAP suicide risk assessment (see Table 5.2 below) could be utilized to help the paramedic assess this.

It is important to note that the patient's account of the events may not reveal the whole picture or be reliable, and it is useful to undertake a holistic history including previous attempts, mental health history and personal circumstances which may be impacting on the patient's mental health. For example, in cases such as personality disorder, the patient may state a high level of suicidal intent, but the circumstances may not appear consistent with this – for instance the overdose has been taken when early detection from family members is likely, or they have themselves called 999. On the other hand, a person may state that they have no intention of suicide, but findings may indicate otherwise such as being alone, they have chosen a time when close family members are away (therefore unlikely to find them) and there is evidence that affairs have been put in order (Hawley et al. 2011).

Self-harm and suicide are growing problems amongst young people. There is a definitive correlation between previous self-harm attempts and future death by suicide, with up to a quarter of patients treated in hospital and returning within one year (Harris et al. 2019). Kapur et al. (2013) believe that effective clinical assessment and management of self-harm can have a positive impact on the outcome, in a patient group who are often considered difficult to help.

Three suicide risk assessment tools that can be used as part of the assessment process are detailed below.

IPAP suicide risk assessment

The IPAP suicide risk assessment tool (see Table 5.2) is a simple tool, adapted for pre-hospital care, which focuses on key areas taken from a range of common UK suicide risk tools. These key areas assess the patient on intent, plan, action and protective measures, and is a structured method to assist with a basic risk assessment. IPAP should be used to help with the management strategy on scene, not as part of long-term condition management. In a mental health context, the risk assessment relates to identifying factors that may indicate a patient who is at higher risk of attempting or completing suicide.

Table 5.2 IPAP suicide risk assessment tool

Intent	Ask the patient if they are currently experiencing thoughts of suicide and explore: • The nature of the thoughts • How often they are experiencing these thoughts • How intrusive the thoughts are
Plan	Has the patient made a plan? While taking the history try to determine: • What is the plan? • Is the plan practical? • Has it been rehearsed? • Does the patient have the means to carry out the plan?
Action	Has any element of the plan been actioned either previously or currently? • If previously – is there a history of mental illness, previous suicide attempts, substance misuse or self-harm? This could indicate a higher risk of completing suicide • Currently – has the patient begun preparations to make a suicide attempt?
Protective measures	Does the patient have any support they can access from: • Family/friends • Mental health services • Local charities

Adapted from AACE and JRCALC (2021)

As with all mental health risk assessment tools, the findings should be used in conjunction with the patient's past and present circumstances, obtaining a full mental and physical health history. If a patient has no support network, they should be deemed to have an increased risk. The IPAP suicide assessment tool can help inform the clinician to devise an appropriate management plan or pathway referral. (See Chapter 8 for further information on pathways.)

The Columbia-Suicide Severity Rating Scale

The Columbia-Suicide Severity Rating Scale (C-SSRS) is a global tool widely used in clinical settings and has been the focus of numerous studies worldwide (Kilincaslan et al. 2019). The tool was initially devised by Columbia University, the University of Pennsylvania and the University of Pittsburgh – supported by the National Institute of Mental Health (NIMH) – to decrease suicide risk among adolescents with depression. The C-SSRS was based on over 20 years of evidence-based study addressing an urgent need for suicide research and prevention.

The scale comprises a series of simple questions measuring suicidal ideations (thoughts of suicide) and behaviours (actions they have taken in preparation for suicide). The amount and choice of questions is dictated by the person's answers, and a severity score is reached which identifies risk and level of support required.

Studies have shown that the scale achieves accurate and comparable results by using consistent, solid psychometric properties (Interian et al. 2018).

Beck Hopelessness Scale

The feeling of hopelessness and depression has a significant correlation with suicidal ideation (McMillan et al. 2007). The Beck Hopelessness Scale (BHS), devised over 40 years ago, is used widely in many countries in primary and secondary care services. The BHS consists of 20 true/false questions relating to feelings about the future, loss of motivation and future expectations. A score of greater than 14 indicates severe hopelessness and the patient may therefore be at risk of suicidal intentions (Kliem et al. 2018). Many of the tools described in this chapter contain elements that relate to feeling desperate or hopeless and it is useful to consider when making an assessment of a patient's risk of suicidal ideation or behaviour.

Substance use

It is important to establish whether a patient undergoing a mental health assessment has consumed alcohol or drugs, as this may pose challenges for the clinician. Many assessment tools contain a question relating to the use of alcohol or drugs – a question also often asked of ambulance clinicians when making a direct referral to a mental health team. This presents challenges, as often when managing the care of patients who require a mental health assessment, paramedics will discover that some level of alcohol consumption has taken place. Although it is accepted that alcohol influences behaviour, whether it will reduce cognitive ability or motor function can be determined by factors such as the quantity consumed. Many mental health services are unable to accept patients who are under the influence of alcohol or drugs as it is part of the admission exclusion criteria. Patients who have used alcohol or drugs may display disruptive, aggressive behaviour and may also have impaired cognitive function (Hawley et al. 2011).

This leaves the paramedic with little alternative other than conveying the patient to an A&E department. However Palmer (2011) suggests that this pathway may not be in the best interests of the patient, particularly if the patient is deemed to have capacity, and proposes that the protocol should be replaced with something less rigid and more flexible, utilizing a 'common-sense' approach.

Assessment in children and adolescents

Children who experience mental health difficulties will usually be referred to the Children and Young People's Mental Health Services (CYPMHS). CYPMHS work alongside other agencies to support children, young people and their families in the assessment and management of a range of mental health conditions (Padmore 2016). Effective communication is particularly important when assessing children and young people to establish the type of support they may require (Kiyimba and O'Reilly 2020).

Child and young person assessment tools

There is a variety of assessment tools used globally in the assessment of children for mental health disorders such as anxiety, obsessive-compulsive disorder, depression, self-harm and suicide risk. Some examples are detailed below.

Strengths and difficulties questionnaire

The strengths and difficulties questionnaire (SDQ) can be used in conjunction with parents or teachers of 4–16 year olds, or as a self-assessment tool for children aged between 11 and 16. Questions cover the type of difficulty the child or young person is experiencing and ascertain the degree of psychological and sociological impact the condition is having on them (Goodman et al. 2009). The questions cover the following areas:

- Emotional symptoms
- Conduct problems
- Hyperactivity/inattention
- Peer relationship problems
- Prosocial behaviour

The tool is considered to be more effective when completed by the child (where appropriate) as well as those who are involved in their care, such as parents, guardians or teachers. Research has shown that early identification of mental health conditions, particularly in children, is essential for healthy cognitive development, and the SDQ can be a useful tool in early assessment (Becker et al. 2015).

Development and Well-Being Assessment

Deighton et al. (2014) believe that the use of patient-reported outcome measures have advantages as they can enhance clinical practice, but conversely, they can be costly and time-consuming to complete. The Development and Well-Being Assessment consists of a series of interviews and questionnaires and is designed to contribute to the formulation of a psychiatric diagnosis. Aimed at 5–17 year olds, it can be completed by the child themselves, parents or teachers. Padmore (2016) advises that this type of assessment can be overwhelming for the child or young person and should be used cautiously, ensuring a clear explanation is given on how it will be conducted and why.

Beck Youth Inventory

The Beck Youth Inventory is a self-reporting tool used for 7–18 year olds to assess mental health conditions such as anxiety and depression, and includes an assessment of anger and disruptive behaviour. The tool is a five-scale inventory containing 20 statements about thoughts, feelings or behaviours associated with emotional and social impairment. Responses to questions are scored as '0' for never and '3' for always, relating to the past two weeks. The Beck Youth Inventory has been adapted over the years and may be used independently or in conjunction with other screening tools (Steer et al. 2001).

Challenges to the mental health assessment

As with any self-assessment tool or questionnaire, the results rely on an individual's responses being accurate. A disadvantage to the mental health assessment tools discussed in this chapter is that results may be affected by a number of factors such as social (if they are being watched while completing the assessment), or personal motivation to overstate or understate severity of symptoms, and they can be time-consuming to undertake. The relationship between the patient and clinician is also an important factor – in order to encourage the patient to share personal experiences, a rapport must be quickly established. In the pre-hospital setting this is challenging due to limited time available to spend with the patient.

The environment in which the patient is being assessed must also be considered. Patients should feel calm and at ease. The ambulance may be the only option for the assessment to take place. This can be a daunting experience for patients who are already in significant distress.

The assessment tool should be simple and well structured in order for the user to fully understand the questions they are being asked. If not used appropriately, they can be nothing more than a 'tick box exercise' (Trenoweth and Moone 2017).

Mental health assessment requires skill: effective communication skills are essential to encourage the patient to respond honestly. Additional training should be given in the use of assessment tools so they can be applied correctly.

As with all assessment tools, clinical judgement, holistic assessment and the clinician's own experience should also be used in the decision-making process.

Risk assessment

The aim of mental health assessment is essentially to determine the level of risk a patient is deemed to be in: current risk of harm and future risk of causing harm to themselves or others. Tools such as the IPAP or C-SSRS will assist in determining suicide risk, but there are other factors to consider. As discussed previously in this chapter, the safety of the clinician is paramount, and measures should be taken to ensure this. Police and other services can be requested to support clinicians at the scene if deemed necessary. If the patient has been using substances such as alcohol or drugs, this can exacerbate symptoms or heighten emotions and paramedics should be aware of the possibility of unpredictable behaviour. Consider any physical risk to the patient such as self-harm or self-neglect, and if their environment is safe for them to be in.

Risk to family or dependants should be assessed, with safeguarding and welfare measures taken where appropriate.

Questions

The use of questions is important in the assessment and history-taking process. Obtaining information from patients who are distressed can be less challenging if a friendly, positive approach is taken. Introduce yourself and always gain consent to ask questions.

Some examples of the types of question used in a mental health assessment are detailed below.

Closed questions

Closed questions can be used to quickly gain facts, and require only short answers. Closed questions also help to keep control of the conversation and maintain focus. For example:

What is your name?
How old are you?
What is your address?
Do you take any medication?
Did you intend to end your own life?

Closed questions may be more appropriate to use with patients who are experiencing concentration difficulties or who are unwilling to engage in conversation.

Open questions

Open questions allow the patient time to think and an opportunity to give you their perspective on the situation. Using open questions can help to avoid missing information that might not be revealed through a closed question.

Can you tell me what has happened today?
How long have you been feeling this way?
Have you ever experienced this before?

Open questions allow the patient to respond in their own way, which may help them to feel at ease.

Probing questions

Probing questions can be used to explore the answers you are given to elicit further information.

What did you want to happen?
Can you explain what you mean?
How often are you experiencing these thoughts?

Clarifying questions

Clarifying what the patient has told you helps to summarize discussions and allows you to pursue greater detail. You may wish to focus on a comment by repeating it back to the patient. Clarifying questions also offer the patient an opportunity for reflection or contemplation. It is also helpful to ensure details have been recorded accurately.

Case study 5.2 History taking

You have been called to a busy pub in a city centre, to a 24 year old woman called Emily. Emily is distressed and has been overheard telling people she wants to end her life. She has bloodstains on her sleeves from recent self-harm attempts.

On arrival you notice that Emily appears unkempt and has two carrier bags with her belongings inside. As you approach Emily, she begins to calm down and walks towards you.

What is your priority?

What information do you need from Emily?

Initial approach: Risk assessment of crew/patient/bystander safety. See Table 5.1 for points to consider during this assessment.

Environment: Is it a suitable environment to assess Emily?

You adopt a calm and friendly approach and ask Emily to speak with you in the back of the ambulance, and she agrees. You gain Emily's consent to ask her some questions and to assess the wounds on her arms.

Emily shows you her arms – she has multiple superficial lacerations which are bleeding, and she consents to treatment.

You undertake a functional test of capacity (see Table 5.2) and decide that Emily has capacity.

You move on to the history taking and mental health assessment. **What questions should you ask Emily? Consider the following factors:**

- A history of any mental health disorder
- A history of any chronic physical health problems
- Any past experience of, and responses to, treatments
- The quality of interpersonal relationships
- Living conditions and social isolation
- A family history of mental illness
- A history of domestic violence or sexual abuse
- Employment and immigration status (NICE 2011)

Emily declares that she is homeless and has a history of previous self-harm, depression and generalized anxiety disorder. **What else do you need to know? What type of questions could you use?**

Consider using a risk assessment tool such as IPAP.

Intent

'Are you experiencing suicidal thoughts now?'
'How long have you been feeling this way?'
'How often are you having suicidal thoughts?'
'Can you describe the thoughts to me?'

Emily tells you she is currently experiencing thoughts of suicide and has been for the past two weeks. She wants to end it all soon as she cannot continue living on the streets.

Plan

'Have you thought about how you are going to end your life?'

'Have you made a plan to carry this out?'
'Have you tried to carry out this plan in the past?' If so, 'When did you make this attempt?'
'Do you think you will kill yourself?'

Consider if Emily's plan is feasible – does she have the means to carry out her plan?

Emily shows you one of her bags, which contains several packets of paracetamol which she has been purchasing every day for the past week, and she tells you she was planning to have several drinks in the pub before taking them all.

Action

Has Emily started to put any plans in place to carry out her plan? Contacted friends/family? Written a note?

Collecting paracetamol would be considered taking action to end her life.

Protective measures

Emily is deemed at higher risk of suicide based on her personal circumstances. Does she have a support network, or contact with mental health workers?

Emily has a couple of friends but no contact with family. She has not seen her key worker for several weeks.

Clarifying questions can help to summarize the current situation:

'Emily, can you confirm to me that you have been experiencing suicidal thoughts regularly for the past two weeks?'
'Have you purchased the paracetamol over the last week with the intention of ending your life today?'

Based on the assessment, Emily is deemed to be at severe risk of suicide and must be seen by a mental health specialist. As Emily has a mental health diagnosis you could consider contacting mental health services via a GP or crisis resolution (see Chapter 8 for pathway referral options). If there are no services available, Emily needs to be taken to A&E for assessment and treatment. All information should be clearly documented and passed on to the receiving clinician.

Conclusion

This chapter has outlined some of the mental health assessment tools used by healthcare professionals and has discussed the importance of undertaking an effective assessment. There are a number of challenges faced by clinicians when assessing a patient with a mental health condition, as highlighted in this chapter, and it is important to consider these. Risk assessments should be undertaken to evaluate risk to the clinician's personal safety as well as patient and bystander safety. A mental capacity assessment should be undertaken on all patients using the functional test of capacity. Taking a history from a distressed patient can be difficult, but adopting a friendly, calm approach using a combination of open, closed and probing questions can assist the clinician in the process. Assessment tools can be utilized as part of the decision-making process but should be used in conjunction with clinical judgement, clinician experience and taking the patient's circumstances into account using a holistic approach.

References

Association of Ambulance Chief Executives (Great Britain) and Joint Royal Colleges Ambulance Liaison Committee (2021) *JRCALC Clinical Guidelines*. Bridgwater: Class Professional Publishing.

Banner, N.F. (2012) Unreasonable reasons: Normative judgements in the assessment of mental capacity, *Journal of Evaluation in Clinical Practice*, 18(5): 1038–44.

Becker, A., Rothenberger, A., Sohn, A., Ravens-Sieberer, U., Klasen, F. and the BELLA study group (2015) Erratum to: Six years ahead: A longitudinal analysis regarding course and predictive value of the Strengths and Difficulties Questionnaire (SDQ) in children and adolescents, *European Child & Adolescent Psychiatry*, 24(6): 727.

Cameron, I.M., Cardy, A., Crawford, J.R. et al. (2011) Measuring depression severity in general practice: Discriminatory performance of the PHQ-9, HADS-D, and BDI-II, *British Journal of General Practice*, 61(588): 419–26.

Cliff, C. and McGraw, C. (2016) The conduct and process of mental capacity assessments in home health care settings, *British Journal of Community Nursing*, 21(11): 570–7.

Deighton, J., Croudace, T., Fonagy, P., Brown, J., Patalay, P. and Wolpert, M. (2014) Measuring mental health and wellbeing outcomes for children and adolescents to inform practice and policy: A review of child self-report measures, *Child and Adolescent Psychiatry and Mental Health*, 8(1): 14.

Goodman, R., Ford, T., Simmons, H., Gatward, R. and Meltzer, H. (2009) Using the Strengths and Difficulties Questionnaire (SDQ) to screen for child psychiatric disorders in a community sample, *International Review of Psychiatry*, 15(1–2): 166–72.

Harris, I.M., Beese, S. and Moore, D. (2019) Predicting future self-harm or suicide in adolescents: A systematic review of risk assessment scales/tools, *BMJ Open*, 9(9): e029311.

Hawley, C., Singhal, A., Roberts, A., Atkinson, H. and Whelan, C. (2011) Mental health in the care of paramedics: part 2, *Journal of Paramedic Practice*, 3(6): 304–12.

Home Office, Public Health England and IOM (2017) *Health Protocol: Pre-Entry Health Assessments For UK-Bound Refugees*. Available at: https://www.england.nhs.uk/south/wp-content/uploads/sites/6/2014/06/refugee-health-protocal.pdf (accessed 21 March 2020).

Interian, A., Chesin, M., Kline, A. et al. (2018) Use of the Columbia-Suicide Severity Rating Scale (C-SSRS) to classify suicidal behaviors, *Archives of Suicide Research*, 22(2): 278–94.

Jones, N. and Greenberg, N. (2015) The use of Threshold Assessment Grid triage (TAG-triage) in mental health assessment, *Journal of the Royal Army Medical Corps*, 161(Suppl1): 46–51.

Kapur, N., Steeg, S., Webb, R. et al. (2013) Does clinical management improve outcomes following self-harm? Results from the Multicentre Study of Self-Harm in England, *PloS One*, 8(8): e70434.

Kilincaslan, A., Gunes, A., Eskin, M. and Madan, A. (2019) Linguistic adaptation and psychometric properties of the Columbia-Suicide Severity Rating Scale among a heterogeneous sample of adolescents in Turkey, *International Journal of Psychiatry in Medicine*, 54(2): 115–32.

Kiyimba, N. and O'Reilly, M. (2020) The clinical use of Subjective Units of Distress scales (SUDs) in child mental health assessments: A thematic evaluation, *Journal of Mental Health*, 29(4): 418–23.

Kliem, S., Lohmann, A., Mößle, T. and Brähler, E. (2018) Psychometric properties and measurement invariance of the Beck hopelessness scale (BHS): Results from a German representative population sample, *BMC Psychiatry*, 18(1): 110.

Levis, B., Benedetti, A. and Thombs, B.D. (2019) Accuracy of Patient Health Questionnaire-9 (PHQ-9) for screening to detect major depression: Individual participant data meta-analysis, *BMJ*, 365: 1476.

Lowthian, J.A., Curtis, A.J., Cameron, P.A., Stoelwinder, J.U., Cooke, M.W. and McNeil, J.J. (2011) Systematic review of trends in emergency department attendances: An Australian perspective, *Emergency Medicine Journal: EMJ*, 28(5): 373–7.

McMillan, D., Gilbody, S., Beresford, E. and Neilly, L. (2007) Can we predict suicide and non-fatal self-harm with the Beck Hopelessness Scale? A meta-analysis, *Psychological Medicine*, 37(6): 769–78.

Mental Capacity Act 2005. Available at: https://www.legislation.gov.uk/ukpga/2005/9/contents (accessed 17 October 2020).

National Institute for Clinical Excellence (NICE) (2004) *Self-Harm: The Short-Term Physical and Psychological Management and Secondary Prevention of Self-Harm in Primary and Secondary Care*. London: NICE (Updated 2018). Available at: https://www.nice.org.uk/guidance/cg16/evidence/full-guideline-189936541 (accessed 30 October 2020).

National Institute for Health and Care Excellence (NICE) (2009) *Depression in Adults: Recognition and Management*. Clinical guideline CG90. Available at: https://www.nice.org.uk/guidance/cg90 (accessed 17 October 2020).

National Institute for Health and Care Excellence (NICE) (2011) *Common Mental Health Problems: Identification and Pathways to Care*. Clinical guideline CG123. Available at: https://www.nice.org.uk/guidance/cg123 (accessed 17 October 2020).

National Institute for Health and Care Excellence (NICE) (2014) *Psychosis and Schizophrenia in Adults: Prevention and Management*. Clinical guideline CG178. Available at: https://www.nice.org.uk/guidance/cg178/chapter/1-recommendations#first-episode-psychosis-2 (accessed 21 September 2020).

Padmore, J. (2016) *The Mental Health Needs of Children and Young People: Guiding You to Key Issues and Practices in CAMHS*. Maidenhead: Open University Press.

Palmer, A. (2011) Improving the assessment and referral of mental health patients, *Journal of Paramedic Practice*, 3(9): 496–503.

Patel, A.S., Harrison, A. and Bruce-Jones, W. (2009) Evaluation of the risk assessment matrix: a mental health triage tool, *Emergency Medicine Journal*, 26(1): 11–14.

Shaban, R. (2006) Paramedics' clinical judgement and mental health assessments in emergency contexts: Research, practice, and tools of the trade, *Australasian Journal of Paramedicine*, 4(2). doi:10.33151/ajp.4.2.369.

Sharma, V.K., Krishna, M., Lepping, P. et al. (2010) Validation and feasibility of the Global Mental Health Assessment Tool – Primary Care Version (GMHAT/PC) in older adults, *Age and Ageing*, 39(4): 496–9.

Slade, M., Powell, R., Rosen, A. and Strathdee, G. (2000) Threshold Assessment Grid (TAG): The development of a valid and brief scale to assess the severity of mental illness, *Social Psychiatry and Psychiatric Epidemiology*, 35(2): 78–85.

Steer, R.A., Kumar, G., Beck, J.S. and Beck, A.T. (2001) Evidence for the construct validities of the Beck Youth Inventories with child psychiatric outpatients, *Psychological Reports*, 89(3): 559–65.

Townsend, E., Ness, J., Waters, K. et al. (2016) Self-harm and life problems: Findings from the Multicentre Study of Self-harm in England, *Social Psychiatry and Psychiatric Epidemiology*, 51(2): 183–92.

Trenoweth, S. and Moone, N. (2017) *Psychosocial Assessment in Mental Health*. Los Angeles: SAGE.

Wright, K. and McGlen, I. (2012) Mental health emergencies: Using a structured assessment framework, *Nursing Standard*, 27(7): 48–56.

Yeager, K. and Roberts, A. (2015) *Crisis Intervention Handbook: Assessment, Treatment, and Research*. Oxford: Oxford University Press.

Further reading

Association of Ambulance Chief Executives (Great Britain) and Joint Royal Colleges Ambulance Liaison Committee (2021) *JRCALC Clinical Guidelines*. Bridgwater: Class Professional Publishing.

Trenoweth, S. and Moone, N. (2017) *Psychosocial Assessment in Mental Health*. Los Angeles: SAGE.

6 Management of complex needs in mental health

Jo Augustus and Yuet Wah Patrick

Learning objectives

- Explore medication concordance specific to commonly prescribed medication for different mental health conditions
- Provide an overview of assessment and treatment pathways for individuals in psychiatric inpatient units
- Outline evidence-based psychosocial interventions
- Discuss treatment pathways for individuals being treated in the community

Introduction

This chapter will explore evidence-based interventions in the assessment and treatment of individuals in different settings. These will include both inpatient and community settings in the context of holistic care provision. The aim is to equip paramedics with appropriate knowledge specific to patient care after the transition to hospital care. Evidence-based interventions will also be discussed with reference to NICE guidelines.

Unconscious bias can influence decision-making processes, therefore it is essential that paramedics have an awareness of their own beliefs while making decisions. Information Box 6.1 addresses this in more detail.

Information box 6.1 Unconscious bias

Unconscious bias is defined as associations or attitudes that automatically change individual perceptions, thus altering behaviour, interactions and decision-making (FitzGerald and Hurst 2017; Marcelin et al. 2019). This may impact on the communication between patient and healthcare provider or the care that is provided (Smedley et al. 2003; Como et al. 2020). A systematic review indicated that unconscious bias affected clinical judgement of both physicians and nurses towards patients. This included bias related to ethnicity, gender, socio-economic status, age, weight, individuals living with HIV, disability, and those who misuse drugs (FitzGerald and Hurst 2017). However, Dehon et al.'s (2017) systematic review found weaker evidence that unconscious bias affected decision-making, specific to race (Marcelin et al. 2019). Subsequently there has been a call to acknowledge unconscious bias and develop strategies to reduce the impact it has in healthcare (Hannah and Carpenter-Song 2013). This impact could include issues pertaining to medication adherence.

Paramedics' unconscious bias could have both a positive and negative impact on patients, for example promoting Making Every Contact Count (MECC), which was devised to empower individuals to make positive behavioural changes, including medication adherence (Public Health England 2016).

Psychosocial factors that influence medication adherence

Pharmacological medication non-adherence is largely about the dosage actually taken, compared to the prescribed dose (Marrero et al. 2020). Pharmacological treatment adherence is an important consideration in relation to the efficacy of treatment (NICE 2009a). Reduced or poor adherence to medication increases the possibility of relapse through symptom deterioration and reduced health benefits, including increased mortality (Simpson et al. 2006; Horne et al. 2013; Marrero et al. 2020). This can also have cost implications for healthcare services through wasted medication and potential increased usage of healthcare (Horne et al. 2013). Adherence can be measured through a variety of different ways, such as self-reporting through questionnaires, including the Medication Adherence Report Scale, Beliefs about Medicines Questionnaire and the Brief Illness Perception Questionnaire (Emilsson et al. 2017). Adherence is not as easily monitored out of hospital and the consequences can often go unnoticed until the person becomes symptomatic. The health belief model was developed as a means to predict health behaviours. Research such as the health belief model has sought to explore factors surrounding non-adherence, as a way to understand changes in individual health behaviours (Rosenstock 1974). This model suggests four elements: susceptibility to illness; severity of illness; barriers to overcoming the illness; and beliefs associated with the effectiveness of treatment. These elements, combined with other factors such as socio-demographics, act to explain health-related behaviours (Marrero et al. 2020).

Paramedics are in a position to gauge medication adherence as they see people in their home environment. Clues such as medication packets that have expired but may be untouched or still contain tablets, or Dossett boxes containing tablets in out-of-sequence days or times, indicate that medication may possibly not be taken as prescribed. It is useful, then, to find out why the person is non-compliant with their medication. Common reasons include:

- forgetfulness, where the person misses a dose (or doses)
- medication fatigue, where they have had enough of taking tablets
- lack of symptoms – the person either feels better and therefore does not see the need to continue taking their medication, or they do not feel any different once they start or stop taking the medication
- concern or worry that they will become addicted to the medication or experience adverse reactions to it
- polypharmacy, where the person becomes confused what medication they should be taking, when and what it is for
- cost, if the person has to pay for their prescriptions

The consequences of non-adherence are deterioration of the condition, increased comorbid conditions, increased hospitalizations and prolonged stays, increased healthcare costs, and even death. Once the reason for non-adherence has been uncovered, the paramedic can signpost or give advice to the person regarding their medication. This upholds the Making Every Contact Count (MECC) initiative launched by Health Education England with the aim of enhancing people's lives by encouraging them to change behaviour for positive health benefits (Public Health England 2016).

Research conducted across a diverse psychiatric population concurs with the health belief model, indicating that adherence is associated with health beliefs in addition to perceptions of barriers to and benefits of the treatment (Marrero et al. 2020). Medication adherence may be seen as less important if symptoms are absent or infrequently occurring (Horne et al. 2013). The patient information provided about the medication may worsen concerns about side effects that outweigh the health benefits, coupled with the perception that medications are overprescribed (Calnan et al. 2005; Bowskill et al. 2007). In addition, worries about dependency, cost and long-term impact are also factors that could influence adherence (Horne et al. 1999; Horne et al. 2013). Research conducted by Emilsson et al. (2017) found that adolescents taking long-term medication for attention deficit hyperactivity disorder (ADHD) had good adherence, that related to beliefs about the necessity to reduce symptoms and less concern about side effects. Non-adherence to ADHD medication can have significant effects across the life course, so beliefs about medication are an important indicator of adherence.

Interventions adapted for different groups and settings can be implemented to improve adherence. Research conducted by McMillan et al. (2018) found that a community pharmacy-based medication support service improved outcomes, such as satisfaction with and adherence to medication. Thus, locally adapted interventions could be effective in addressing the issues surrounding non-adherence (NICE 2009a). Horne et al. (2013) proposes adopting a patient-centred model of communication that encompasses the patient's perception, resolving concerns and increasing the convenience of the medication. Thus, interventions that encompass patients' views through delivery of patient-centred care are seen as essential to improving medication adherence.

The following sections will explore medication using the structure of medication types, side-effects and contraindicators.

Selective serotonin reuptake inhibitors

Selective serotonin reuptake inhibitors (SSRIs) are used in the treatment of depression and can also be used to treat other mental health conditions such as anxiety disorders and bulimia (NICE 2021). Table 6.1 summarizes commonly prescribed SSRIs.

Table 6.1 Selective serotonin reuptake inhibitors

Commonly prescribed medication/initial dosage	Commonly experienced side effects
Sertraline 50mg Fluoxetine 20mg Citalopram 20mg Escitalopram 10mg Paroxetine 20mg	**Common** anxiety; appetite abnormal; arrhythmias; arthralgia; asthenia; concentration impaired; confusion; constipation; depersonalization; diarrhoea; dizziness; drowsiness; dry mouth; fever; gastrointestinal discomfort; haemorrhage; headache; hyperhidrosis; malaise; memory loss; menstrual cycle irregularities; myalgia; mydriasis; nausea (dose-related); palpitations; paraesthesia; QT interval prolongation; sexual dysfunction; skin reactions; sleep disorders; taste altered; tinnitus; tremor; urinary disorders; visual impairment; vomiting; weight changes; yawning **Uncommon** alopecia; angioedema; behaviour abnormal; hallucination; mania; movement disorders; photosensitivity reaction; postural hypotension; seizure; suicidal behaviours; syncope

Adapted from NICE (2021)

Contraindicators: SSRIs

Cardiac disease; concurrent electroconvulsive therapy; diabetes mellitus; epilepsy (discontinue if convulsions develop); history of bleeding disorders (especially gastrointestinal bleeding); history of mania; susceptibility to angle-closure glaucoma.

Medications that can interact with some SSRIs include:

- **non-steroidal anti-inflammatory drugs (NSAIDs)** – a common type of painkiller that includes ibuprofen
- **antiplatelets** – a type of medication used to prevent blood clots, such as low-dose aspirin and clopidogrel (NICE 2021)

Antipsychotic medication

Antipsychotic medications are used to treat symptoms of psychosis, including seeing and hearing things that other people cannot see or hear. They are classified into first-generation (typical) and second-generation (atypical) antipsychotics. First-generation antipsychotics are thought to block dopamine D2 receptors in the brain and second-generation antipsychotics act on a variety of receptors (NICE 2021). Table 6.2 summarizes commonly prescribed antipsychotic medications.

Table 6.2 Antipsychotic medications

Commonly prescribed medication/dosage	Common side effects
Quetiapine 600mg Risperidone 4–6mg Olanzapine 15mg Aripiprazole 15mg Haloperidol 8mg	**Common** agitation; amenorrhoea; arrhythmias; constipation; dizziness; drowsiness; dry mouth; galactorrhoea; gynaecomastia; hyperprolactinaemia; hypotension; insomnia; leucopenia; movement disorders; neutropenia; parkinsonism; QT interval prolongation; rash; seizure; tremor; urinary retention; vomiting **Uncommon** agranulocytosis; confusion; embolism and thrombosis; neuroleptic malignant syndrome

Adapted from NICE (2021)

Contraindicators: antipsychotic medication

Blood dyscrasias; cardiovascular disease; conditions predisposing to seizures; depression; diabetes; epilepsy; history of jaundice; myasthenia gravis; Parkinson's disease; photosensitization; prostatic hypertrophy; severe respiratory disease.

NB: An ECG may be required, particularly if physical examination identifies cardiovascular risk factors, personal history of cardiovascular disease, or if the patient is being admitted as an inpatient.

Medication and mental health conditions

Depression

Depression is largely treated in primary care, however some individuals made need emergency care, with particular reference to severe presentations. This may include individuals who present with an increased risk of harm to self, including suicidal ideation, high levels of self-neglect and/or the presence of psychotic features. In addition, comorbidity including physical heath and/or mental health conditions may feature. Dual diagnosis may also be present where the use of drugs or alcohol features. Triggers may include loss and change, for example death of a loved one, loss of job, divorce (WHO 2018). SSRIs can be prescribed by a GP or psychiatrist, but these can take two to three months to start working (see Table 6.1). Benzodiazepine (e.g. diazepam) can be prescribed for more immediate relief of anxiety symptoms, typically taking up to 1.5 hours to work.

Anxiety disorders

Similar to depression, anxiety disorders are largely treated and managed in primary care by GPs. However, some individuals may present to emergency services with panic attacks, characterized by an isolated episode of intense fear or apprehension with the sudden onset of symptoms including heart palpitations or an increased heart rate (WHO 2018). Panic attacks can be experienced as a random occurrence or triggered by a situation. In addition, panic disorder is the reoccurrence of panic attacks not limited to particular situations or stimuli. They may also include the catastrophic misinterpretation of symptoms, such as the belief that the individual is having a heart attack. Panic attacks usually dissipate within a few minutes and if they frequently reoccur referral to the GP may be appropriate. Medication is usually SSRIs and/or benzodiazepines.

Disorders due to substance use

These include disorders, including single episodes of substance use that result in harm, due to misuse of substances including, but not limited to, alcohol, opioids and hallucinogens. This can lead to substance-induced disorders such as substance withdrawal and substance-induced mental disorders, sexual dysfunction and sleep-wake disorders (WHO 2018). Treatment is usually a combination of medication and psychosocial interventions.

Table 6.3 outlines substances that are commonly abused and how an individual may present.

Table 6.3   Disorders due to substance use

Substance	Presentation
Alcohol	Dysarthria, poor coordination, ataxia, nystagmus, diplopia, impaired memory and drowsiness, behavioural outbursts
Cannabis	Initially euphoric, afterwards drowsy, increased appetite, conjunctival injection, dry mouth, tachycardia and paranoia
Amphetamines, methamphetamine or methcathinone	Euphoria, excitement, arousal, agitation, dilatation of pupils, tachycardia or bradycardia, hypertension or hypotension, repetitive motor movements, paranoia, confusion, seizures and coma
MDMA or related drugs, including MDA	Similar to, but less potent than, amphetamine, excessive feelings of belonging and/or closeness, dehydration, hyperthermia
Opiates	Initially euphoric, afterwards drowsy, constricted pupils, slurred speech and poor concentration
Sedatives, hypnotics or anxiolytics	Dysarthria, poor coordination, ataxia, nystagmus, diplopia, sedation, impaired memory

Adapted from NICE (2021) and WHO (2018)

Alcohol withdrawal

Delirium tremens is considered a medical emergency, characterized by agitation, confusion, paranoia, and visual and auditory hallucinations. Oral lorazepam should be used as a first-line treatment (NICE 2021).

Opiate withdrawal

Opiate withdrawal is not generally considered a medical emergency. It is characterized by nausea/vomiting, myalgia, lacrimation, running nose, diarrhoea, sweating, yawning, insomnia and fever. Methadone or buprenorphine can be prescribed under supervision to assist withdrawal.

Schizophrenia

Schizophrenia is characterized by disturbances in multiple mental modalities – e.g. delusions and/or disorganization in thinking (WHO 2018). Once an initial risk assessment has been completed, the individual can be treated with antipsychotics by a psychiatrist (see Table 6.2). As part of emergency medicine, tranquilization may need to be a consideration for the psychiatrists. An assessment under the Mental Health Act may need to be completed.

Bipolar disorder

Bipolar disorder is an episodic mood disorder characterized by the occurrence of manic, mixed or hypomanic episodes or symptoms. Such episodes usually alternate over the course of these disorders with depressive episodes or depressive symptoms (WHO 2018). Bipolar disorder can be treated with antipsychotics lithium, valproate or lamotrigine (see Table 6.2). Psychological therapy may also be recommended.

Information box 6.2 Toxicity: lithium

Lithium as a psychiatric intervention dates back to the mid-nineteenth century and was reintroduced in 1949 for the treatment of mania (Shorter 2009). In contemporary psychiatry lithium is prescribed for the treatment and prophylaxis of mania, bipolar disorder, recurrent depression and aggressive or self-harming behaviour (NICE 2021). However, within the typical therapeutic range of 0.4–1.0mmol/l close monitoring is required to actively prevent toxicity from occurring (Baird-Gunning et al. 2017; Foulser et al. 2017).

Table 6.4　Lithium toxicity

Acute lithium toxicity	nausea, vomiting, diarrhoea, dysrhythmia and neurological manifestations such as coarse tremor, muscle weakness, cerebellar signs and delirium
Severe lithium toxicity	seizures, coma and permanent neurological effects such as dementia

Adapted from Foulser et al. (2017)

The effects of lithium toxicity are summarized in Table 6.4. Lithium toxicity can include multiple systems and manifest in a variety of different presentations. In the context of emergency medicine, patients prescribed lithium and presenting with the above symptoms should have their lithium levels checked immediately. Lithium levels that are above 1.2mmol/l are of immediate clinical concern (NICE 2021).

Anorexia nervosa

Anorexia nervosa is characterized by significantly low body weight for the individual's height, age and developmental stage. Other health conditions need to be ruled out, and recognition of the availability of food needs to be established. A commonly used threshold is a body mass index (BMI) of less than 18.5 kg/m^2 in adults (WHO 2018). Individuals with a historic or current diagnosis of anorexia nervosa may present with physical health symptoms or comorbid mental health difficulties such as depression. Therefore, once a risk assessment has been completed patients considered high risk should be transported to hospital for further assessment. A mental health assessment may need to be completed. Medication should be prescribed in conjunction with other interventions, such as counselling.

Postnatal or antenatal depression

Postnatal or antenatal depression associated with pregnancy or puerperium is characterized by significant mental and behavioural features, most commonly depressive symptoms (WHO 2018). This can be with or without the presence of delusions, hallucinations or other psychotic symptoms. Postnatal or antenatal depression in a mild presentation can be managed in primary care and treated by a combination of medication and psychosocial interventions. However, severe presentations where neglect or suicidal ideation is present may require immediate psychiatric assessment and possible admission. Paramedics may need to follow the local safeguarding policy to seek guidance.

Acute behavioural disturbance (ABD)

Although not a term used in diagnostic criteria, acute behavioural disturbance is used to describe the clinical presentation of different conditions that usually constitute a medical emergency and require transfer to the emergency department without delay. This will increase the success of treatment being provided. These conditions include, but are not limited to, psychiatric disorders, sepsis, substance misuse, head injury or seizure, neuroleptic malignant syndrome, thyroid storm, heat exhaustion and dementia.

Patients should be taken to the nearest emergency department if they exhibit the following:

- tactile hyperthermia
- constant or near constant physical activity, without exhaustion
- extreme agitation/aggression (The Royal College of Emergency Medicine 2019)

Information box 6.3 Stigma and antidepressants

Stigma specific to the treatment of depression can act as a barrier to individuals accessing evidence-based interventions (Schnyder et al. 2017; Kelly et al. 2019). This can have negative implications for the individual, their family and carers, so it is important to acknowledge this in order to challenge such beliefs and attitudes. Research conducted by Kelly et al. (2019) found that although stigma specific to depression was reducing, attitudes towards antidepressants remained negative, especially in men. Schnyder et al. (2017) reported that a negative attitude towards one's own and others' mental health difficulties acted as a barrier to help-seeking behaviours.

Psychological therapy intervention

This section explores psychological interventions in more detail.

Therapy versus pharmacology

As part of evidence-based practice, pharmacology and psychological therapies are recognized as effective treatments for a variety of mental health difficulties. For many mild to moderate mental health diagnoses psychological therapy is recommended as a first-line intervention, followed by medication, whereas for severe and enduring diagnoses medication is offered as a first-line intervention. However, research has shown that this is dependent on multiple factors, including, but not limited to, patient history and diagnosis. Interventions should also be implemented as the least intrusive first-line intervention, which is in line with the stepped model of care (see Figure 6.1).

Figure 6.1 Stepped care model

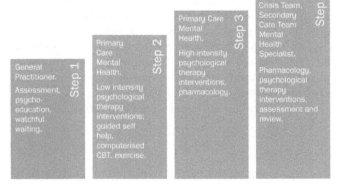

Adapted from NICE (2009a; 2011)

The stepped care model consists of a range of interventions, beginning with low-intensity psychological interventions, that might include attendance at psycho-educational groups, self-help and guided self-help interventions, for milder presentations. High-intensity psychological interventions may include individual cognitive behaviour therapy or pharmacology intervention. Those with more complex presentations may require highly specialized treatment delivered by a multidisciplinary team in the community or an inpatient setting. This may include pharmacology and/or psychological treatment (NICE 2011). It is of great importance that a person-centred approach, with shared decision-making, is taken, where there is an emphasis on accessible information about the available options. This will act to support the improvement of patient outcomes (Adams and Drake 2006; Raphael et al. 2021).

There has been extensive research conducted over the years exploring the effectiveness of interventions in order to establish the most effective first-line intervention. The following will briefly explore this in relation to depression and anxiety, in line with NICE guidance recommendations (Augustus et al. 2019).

Depression

For mild to moderate depression first-line interventions may include self-help programmes, computerized cognitive behaviour therapy and physical exercise programmes (NICE 2009b). Antidepressant medication would not usually be considered for mild depression, however it may be for moderate symptoms. For moderate to severe depression, antidepressant medication and psychological therapy should be offered. Therapy could be either cognitive behaviour therapy or interpersonal therapy. Risk assessments are conducted as routine practice. Additional support can be considered through referral to specialist mental health services (NICE 2009b).

Anxiety

For individuals experiencing mild to moderate anxiety, interventions may include psycho-educational groups, self-help or guided self-help. Moderate to severe presentations are usually offered a choice of cognitive behaviour therapy or pharmacology. For individuals with severe presentations a highly specialist approach should be taken that includes pharmacology and/or psychological interventions. This can be delivered in the community by the crisis team, for example, or as part of inpatient care (NICE 2011).

Children and Young People's Mental Health Services

The GP usually refers children and young people to specialist Children and Young People's Mental Health Services (CYPMHS) for assessment. CYPMHS is a multidisciplinary service involving a variety of different mental health specialists, such as mental health nurses, occupational therapists and psychologists (O'Reilly et al. 2019). The assessment includes diagnosis and treatment as appropriate, for children and young people experiencing difficulties associated with emotional, behavioural or neurodevelopmental disorders (Karim 2015). Family and/or carers may be involved in the assessment, and in some instances the treatment process, to provide information and help support the child's progress. In addition, family therapy may also be a recommended treatment (Karim 2015).

There are similarities in the recommended evidence-based interventions for both adults and children and young people, as outlined in NICE guidelines. Such similarities include psychosocial and pharmacological interventions for certain diagnoses. For example, in the management of mild depression, watchful waiting and psychological therapies may be suggested (NICE 2019). The treatment of psychosis and schizophrenia may also involve both psychosocial and pharmacological interventions (NICE 2016). However, there is an emphasis on not prescribing antipsychotic medication if symptoms are not sufficient for a diagnosis of psychosis and schizophrenia. Similarly, children and young people with antisocial behaviour and conduct disorder should not be offered pharmacological interventions in routine management unless their behaviour is severely aggressive or coexists with ADHD (NICE 2017).

Inpatient settings

If an individual is admitted formally or informally to an inpatient unit, the treatment outlined above should also be routinely offered. Raphael et al. (2021) recognize that the biomedical model can dominate care provision, however research has found that psychosocial interventions can support the improvement of symptoms (Paterson et al. 2018). Such interventions include structured and semi-structured activities with the intention of supporting the individual to work towards their recovery journey. This may include evidence-based psychological therapies delivered either individually or in a group. Interventions may also be activity-based, such as gardening, walking or day trips. While the intention is to help alleviate symptoms associated with the mental health diagnosis, this may also help support social functioning and integration to help prepare the individual for discharge. However, the suitability of these activities would need to be risk assessed on a case-by-case basis. At the point of admission, the individual should be offered an assessment as part of their care plan that includes collaboratively identifying the most appropriate psychosocial intervention. Lomas et al. (2015) reported that patients were more likely to engage if given a choice of intervention. Furthermore, Molin et al. (2016) stipulated that interventions acting to manage symptoms and seeking to empower patients or offer them hope are also more likely to be well attended. Engagement in such activities is routinely reviewed as part of ward rounds, which usually occur weekly (Raphael et al. 2021).

Information box 6.4 Terminology specific to suicide

The language used to describe events can often fuel stigma and a sense of shame. For example, a phrase such as 'committed suicide', which emerged in some historical contexts, insinuates that a crime has been committed. In some countries and religions, suicide was regarded as a reportable offence (Sommer-Rotenberg 1998; Silverman 2006). In some contemporary societies suicide is seen as a selfish act that neglects to consider the impact on others. While bereavement brings with it stages of grief, this can be exacerbated by a further sense of guilt and shame after suicide. Therefore, by replacing these terms with alternatives such as 'death by suicide' or 'non-fatal suicide attempt' it is hoped to reduce the stigma and shame, replacing it with the opportunity for a healthy discourse (Sommer-Rotenberg 1998).

Assessment and treatment pathways: community

This section will describe referral pathways that are available and the patient's journey, with the aim of helping the decision-making process. When adopting the interdisciplinary approach, an awareness of the roles and responsibilities of those involved in the recovery journey is important to enable the paramedic to make the right referral. Challenges in making the right referral are increased as a result of a reduction in service provision due to lack of funding, the presence of exclusion criteria (for example, substance misuse) and a knowledge gap of the roles of other professionals involved in the recovery journey.

Currently, paramedics are not equipped with the knowledge or training to conduct an assessment of the person's mental health, so their role lies in assessing the person's physical health, providing necessary medical treatment and referring them on to someone who can help them with their mental health. However, getting the right care to someone experiencing a mental health crisis in the pre-hospital environment is particularly challenging due to the limited services that are available to assess them, especially during 'out of office hours'. This has resulted in a number of inappropriate emergency department admissions as there were no other suitable alternatives enabling the person to be assessed. This is reflected in the findings of a survey which discovered that only 14 per cent of adults surveyed felt they were provided with the right response when in crisis, and only half of community teams were able to offer an adequate 24-hour, seven-day crisis service (CQC 2015).

In light of the current COVID-19 pandemic, it is anticipated that the number of people needing mental health support will be unprecedented, leading to additional demand on an already overstretched health service. An improved system including multidisciplinary strategies must be implemented to meet the growing demands of mental health crises.

The Keogh Review recognized the importance in developing round the clock community mental health services, as it states that one of the key changes needed to take place to deliver an improved urgent and emergency service is:

> Providing responsive, urgent physical and mental health services outside of hospital every day of the week, so people no longer choose to queue in hospital emergency departments …

> Patients in mental health crisis ideally should be conveyed to 24/7 mental health referral assessment units, including health-based Section 136 suite/ place of safety. (Urgent and Emergency Care Review Programme Team 2015)

NICE (2020) supports multidisciplinary strategies where ambulance trusts, emergency departments and mental health trusts work in partnership to develop locally agreed protocols for ambulance staff to consider alternative care pathways to emergency departments for people who have self-harmed, where this is appropriate and does not increase the risks to the service user. Primary care, acute and mental health trusts should consider the level of support needed for the delivery of an adequate pre-hospital care system for self-harm.

> Specific consideration should be given to the provision of telephone advice to ambulance staff from crisis resolution teams, approved social workers and Section 12 approved doctors, regarding the assessment of mental capacity and the possible use of the Mental Health Act in the urgent assessment of people who have self-harmed. (NICE 2020)

The NHS (2019) long-term plan echoed the benefits of a multidisciplinary team offering round the clock services and promised:

- 24/7 community-based mental health crisis response for adults and older adults across England by 2020/21 offering intensive home treatment as an alternative to an acute inpatient admission.
- A single point of access and timely, universal mental health crisis care for everyone, with 24/7 access in the community, will be provided over the next ten years.
- Alternative forms of provision for those experiencing mental health crisis will be set up such as sanctuaries, safe havens and crisis cafes. These will provide a more suitable alternative to A&E for many people, usually for people whose needs are escalating to crisis point, or who are experiencing a crisis, but do not necessarily have medical needs that require A&E admission.
- 24/7 age-appropriate crisis service for children and young people. This will include a comprehensive offer of crisis assessment, brief follow-up and intensive home treatment.

A dedicated national investment programme to improve the capacity of the ambulance service to meet mental health needs has also been introduced in response to the NHS (2019) long-term plan. This will include:

- funding for mental health professionals in ambulance control rooms to improve telephone triage and support, avoiding conveyance to emergency departments where appropriate
- a national programme to increase mental health training and education of ambulance staff
- (subject to the Capital Spending Review) funding for dedicated mental health response vehicles (and staff) to increase capacity to respond in a more timely manner, and in a more suitable vehicle (see street triage in Table 6.5)

Table 6.5 summarizes some of the care pathways that are available to paramedics when they are dealing with a person in crisis. Protocols and services differ in separate localities so the paramedic should follow local procedure when making referrals.

Table 6.5   Summary of care pathways

Service	Description
Mental health professional in ambulance control room	Mental health professionals, such as a mental health nurse, offer specialist advice and support to ambulance staff caring for patients with mental ill health or substance misuse issues. They help triage patients, identifying what support is needed, and facilitate referrals to appropriate services.
	A six-month pilot in the Yorkshire Ambulance Service NHS Trust showed that 48 per cent of mental health calls were usually conveyed to emergency departments, but this reduced to 18 per cent when triaged by a mental health nurse (NHS 2019).
Street triage	Several ambulance trusts have adopted, or are piloting, the street triage scheme, which consists of a paramedic working in partnership with a police officer and a mental health specialist who respond to mental health crisis calls. Between them, they can assess the person's mental and physical health, signpost and make the appropriate referrals including detention under s136 if necessary.
	Early results from street triage show that s136 detentions have reduced, as have the number of emergency department admissions for mental health crisis.
Emergency department	There are times when it is appropriate to convey a person in crisis to ED as they need immediate medical attention. Red flag criteria (see Table 6.6) give the paramedic guidance on what to consider as appropriate for emergency department admission. The list is not exhaustive and the paramedic should be guided by their judgement if the person has other conditions that need emergency department attention.
Crisis Resolution and Home Treatment (CRHT) team	The Crisis Resolution and Home Treatment (CRHT) team is made up of mental health professionals such as a psychiatrist, mental health nurses, social workers and support workers, who offer support to people who are usually already under their care. The care they provide ranges from self-help techniques, community visits, medication administration and assessment of needs. Not all crisis teams operate 24/7 so paramedics are advised to familiarize themselves with local teams for their times of service.
Key worker	People who have already had contact with a mental health service may have been assigned a key worker who works closely with them to support the individual to be able to live in the community. It may be possible for the key worker to be contacted for advice or for them to visit in times of crisis.

(Continued)

Service	Description
GP	Emergency appointments can be made so the person is seen on the same day if they are experiencing a crisis that is not appropriate for emergency department admission.
Helplines	There are a number of organizations and charities that operate helplines where a trained listener will give support to the person in crisis. While they are not usually mental health specialists who can assess people for appropriate referrals, often a listening ear is all the person needs, dismissing the need for further services at that time.
Family and friends	The biggest support a person can have comes from their family and friends. If a person is in crisis but is well enough to stay at home until services are available (e.g. GP appointment, key worker visit), it is reassuring to know that family and friends can be with them until they are seen.

Table 6.6 outlines red flags, including notable serious physical signs.

Table 6.6 Summary of red flag criteria

Red flag criteria (not an exhaustive list) – police/paramedic triggers for conditions requiring treatment or assessment in an emergency department

Dangerous mechanisms:	Serious physical signs:
Patient has:	Noisy breathing
	Not rousable to verbal commands
• been hit by a taser	Suspected fractures
• significant blows to the body	Deep cuts
• fallen > 4 feet	
• injury from edged or projectile weapon	Head injuries:
• been exposed to throttling/ strangulation	• loss of consciousness at any time
• been hit by a vehicle	• facial swelling
• been ejected from a moving vehicle	• bleeding from nose or ears
• been a passenger of a vehicle involved in a collision	
• taken or suspected to have taken drugs or an overdose	
Actual (current) attempt of self-harm:	Possible excited delirium
	Two or more from:
• actively head banging	
• actual use of edged blade to self-harm	• serious physical resistance/ abnormal strength
• ligature use	• high body temperature

(Continued)

Table 6.6 (Continued)

Red flag criteria (not an exhaustive list) – police/paramedic triggers for conditions requiring treatment or assessment in an emergency department	
• evidence of overdose or poisoning • psychiatric crisis (with self-harm) • delusions/hallucinations • mania	• profuse sweating or hot skin • removal of clothing • behavioural confusion/coherence • bizarre behaviour
At the request of ambulance staff, a senior clinician may be requested to perform advanced interventions where the journey would involve too much risk, either to the patient, paramedic or police officer without it.	Conveyance to the nearest emergency department should **not** be undertaken in a police vehicle under any circumstances where a **red flag** trigger is involved.

Adapted from The Royal College of Emergency Medicine (2017)

Referral pathways for mental health crisis vary depending on the services available and the presenting crisis. Figure 6.2 gives an example of pathways that may be followed in the out-of-hospital setting. Deviations from this will occur according to guidance from local policies and service availability.

Figure 6.2 Example of an ambulance referral pathway

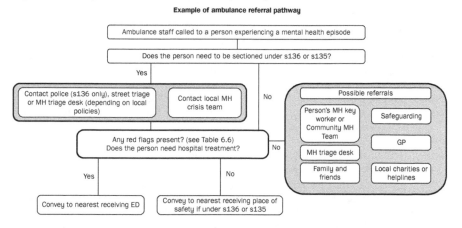

Example of ambulance referral pathway

Conclusion

This chapter has explored a variety of bio-psycho-social interventions in the management of complex mental health needs. The focus has been on evidence-based practice correct at the time of writing, however the authors recognize that research is ever-evolving and therefore interventions may change over time.

References

Adams, J.R. and Drake, R.E. (2006) Shared decision-making and evidence-based practice, *Community Mental Health Journal*, 42(1): 87–105.

Augustus, J., Bold, J. and Williams, B. (2019) *An Introduction to Mental Health*. London: Sage.

Baird-Gunning, J., Lea-Henry, T., Hoegberg, L.C.G., Gosselin, S. and Roberts, D.M. (2017) Lithium poisoning, *Journal of Intensive Care Medicine*, 32: 249–63. doi:10.1177/0885066616651582.

Bowskill, R., Clatworthy, J., Parham, R., Rank, T. and Horne, R. (2007) Patients' perceptions of information received about medication prescribed for bipolar disorder: Implications for informed choice, *Journal of Affective Disorders*, 100(1–3): 253–7.

Calnan, M., Montaner, D. and Horne, R. (2005) How acceptable are innovative health-care technologies? A survey of public beliefs and attitudes in England and Wales, *Social Science & Medicine*, 60(9): 1937–48.

Care Quality Commission (CQC) (2015) *Right Here Right Now: People's Experiences of Help, Care and Support during a Mental Health Crisis*. Newcastle upon Tyne: CQC. Available at: https://www.cqc.org.uk/sites/default/files/20150630_righthere_mhcrisis-care_full.pdf (accessed 30 May 2021).

Como, D.H., Floríndez, L.I., Tran, C.F., Cermak, S.A. and Stein Duker, L.I. (2020) Examining unconscious bias embedded in provider language regarding children with autism, *Nursing & Health Sciences*, 22(2): 197–204.

Dehon, E., Weiss, N., Jones, J., Faulconer, W., Hinton, E. and Sterling, S. (2017) A systematic review of the impact of physician implicit racial bias on clinical decision making, *Academic Emergency Medicine*, 24(8): 895–904.

Emilsson, M., Gustafsson, P.A., Öhnström, G. and Marteinsdottir, I. (2017) Beliefs regarding medication and side effects influence treatment adherence in adolescents with attention deficit hyperactivity disorder, *European Child and Adolescent Psychiatry*, 26(5): 559–71.

FitzGerald, C. and Hurst, S. (2017) Implicit bias in healthcare professionals: A systematic review, *British Medical Council Medical Ethics*, 18(1): 19.

Foulser, P., Abbasi, Y., Mathilakath, A. and Nilforooshan, R. (2017) Do not treat the numbers: Lithium toxicity, *BMJ Case Reports*, 2017: bcr-2017-220079.

Hannah, S.D. and Carpenter-Song, E. (2013) Patrolling your blind spots: Introspection and public catharsis in a medical school faculty development course to reduce unconscious bias in medicine, *Culture, Medicine and Psychiatry*, 37(2): 314–39.

Horne, R., Weinman, J. and Hankins, M. (1999) The Beliefs about Medicines Questionnaire: The development and evaluation of a new method for assessing the cognitive representation of medication, *Psychology and Health*, 14(1): 1–24.

Horne, R., Chapman, S.C.E., Parham, R., Freemantle, N., Forbes, A. and Cooper, V. (2013) Understanding patients' adherence-related beliefs about medicines prescribed for long-term conditions: A meta-analytic review of the Necessity-Concerns Framework, *PloS One*, 8(12): e80633.

Karim, K. (2015) The value of conversation analysis: A child psychiatrist's perspective, in M. O'Reilly and J.N. Lester (eds) *The Palgrave Handbook of Child Mental Health: Discourse and Conversation Studies*. Basingstoke: Palgrave Macmillan, pp. 25–41.

Kelly, J.R., Cosgrove, M., Judd, C., Scott, K., Loughlin, A.M. and O'Keane, V. (2019) Mood matters: A national survey on attitudes to depression, *Irish Journal of Medical Science*, 188(4): 1317–27.

Lomas, T., Cartwright, T., Edginton, T. and Ridge, D. (2015) A qualitative analysis of experiential challenges associated with meditation practice, *Mindfulness*, 6(4): 848–60.

Marcelin, J.R., Siraj, D.S., Victor, R., Kotadia, S. and Maldonado, Y.A. (2019) The impact of unconscious bias in healthcare: How to recognize and mitigate it, *Journal of Infectious Diseases*, 220(Supp2): S62–S73.

Marrero, R.J., Fumero, A., de Miguel, A. and Peñate, W. (2020) Psychological factors involved in psychopharmacological medication adherence in mental health patients: A systematic review, *Patient Education and Counseling*, 103(10): 2116–31.

McMillan, S.S., Kelly, F., Hattingh, H.L., Fowler, J.L., Mihala, G. and Wheeler, A.J. (2018) The impact of a person-centred community pharmacy mental health medication support service on consumer outcomes, *Journal of Mental Health*, 27(2): 164–73.

Molin, J., Graneheim, U.H. and Lindgren, B. (2016) Quality of interactions influences everyday life in psychiatric inpatient care – patients' perspectives, *International Journal of Qualitative Studies on Health and Well-Being*, 11(1): 29897.

NHS (2019) *The NHS Long Term Plan*. Available at: https://www.longtermplan.nhs.uk/wp-content/uploads/2019/08/nhs-long-term-plan-version-1.2.pdf (accessed 30 May 2021).

National Institute for Health and Care Excellence (NICE) (2009a) *Medicines Adherence: Involving Patients in Decisions about Prescribed Medicines and Supporting Adherence*. Clinical guideline CG76. Available at: https://www.nice.org.uk/guidance/cg76 (accessed 25 May 2021).

National Institute for Health and Care Excellence (NICE) (2009b) *Depression in Adults: Recognition and Management*. Clinical guideline CG90. Available at: https://www.nice.org.uk/guidance/cg90 (accessed 25 May 2021).

National Institute for Health and Care Excellence (NICE) (2011) *Generalised Anxiety Disorder and Panic Disorder in Adults: Management*. Clinical guideline CG113. Available at: https://www.nice.org.uk/guidance/cg113 (accessed 25 May 2021).

National Institute for Health and Care Excellence (NICE) (2016) *Psychosis and Schizophrenia in Children and Young People: Recognition and Management*. Clinical guideline CG155. London: NICE.

National Institute for Health and Care Excellence (NICE) (2017) *Antisocial Behaviour and Conduct Disorders in Children and Young People: Recognition and Management*. Clinical guideline CG158. London: NICE.

National Institute for Health and Care Excellence (NICE) (2019) *Depression in Children and Young People: Identification and Management*. NICE guideline NG134. London: NICE.

National Institute for Health and Care Excellence (NICE) (2020) *Initial Management of Self-Harm by Ambulance Staff*. Available at: https://webcache.googleusercontent.com/search?q=cache:6Niby7ue5RcJ:https://pathways.nice.org.uk/pathways/self-harm/initial-management-of-self-harm-by-ambulance-staff.pdf+&cd=1&hl=en&ct=clnk&gl=uk (accessed 30 May 2021).

National Institute for Health and Care Excellence (NICE) (2021) *BNF*. Available at: https://bnf.nice.org.uk (accessed 15 May 2021).

O'Reilly, M., Kiyimba, N. and Nina Lester, J. (2019) Building a case for accessing service provision in child and adolescent mental health assessments, *Discourse Studies*, 21(4): 421–37.

Paterson, C., Karatzias, T., Dickson, A., Harper, S., Dougall, N. and Hutton, P. (2018) Psychological therapy for inpatients receiving acute mental health care: A systematic review and meta-analysis of controlled trials, *British Journal of Clinical Psychology*, 57(4): 453–72.

Public Health England (2016) *Making Every Contact Count (MECC): Consensus Statement*. London: Public Health England. Available at: https://assets.publishing.service.

gov.uk/government/uploads/system/uploads/attachment_data/file/769486/Making_ Every_Contact_Count_Consensus_Statement.pdf (accessed 1 June 2021).

Raphael, J., Price, O., Hartley, S., Haddock, G., Bucci, S. and Berry, K. (2021) Overcoming barriers to implementing ward-based psychosocial interventions in acute inpatient mental health settings: A meta-synthesis, *International Journal of Nursing Studies*, 115(1): 103870.

Rosenstock, I.M. (1974) Historical origins of the health belief model, *Health Education Monographs*, 2(4): 328–35.

Schnyder, N., Panczak, R., Groth, N. and Schultze-Lutter, F. (2017) Association between mental health-related stigma and active help-seeking: Systematic review and meta-analysis, *British Journal of Psychiatry*, 210(4): 261–8.

Shorter E. (2009) The history of lithium therapy, *Bipolar Disorders*, 11(Supp2): 4–9. https://doi.org/10.1111/j.1399-5618.2009.00706.x

Silverman, M.M. (2006) The language of suicidology, *Suicide & Life-Threatening Behaviour*, 36(5): 519–32.

Simpson, S.H., Eurich, D.T., Majumdar, S.R. et al. (2006) A meta-analysis of the association between adherence to drug therapy and mortality, *BMJ*, 333: 15.

Smedley, B.D., Stith, A.Y. and Nelson, A.R. (2003) *Unequal Treatment: Confronting Racial and Ethnic Disparities in Healthcare*. Washington, DC: National Academy Press.

Sommer-Rotenberg, D. (1998) Suicide and language, *Canadian Medical Association Journal*, 159(3): 239–40.

The Royal College of Emergency Medicine (2017) *A Brief Guide to Section 136 for Emergency Departments*. London: Royal College of Emergency Medicine. Available at: https://www.rcem.ac.uk/docs/College%20Guidelines/A%20brief%20guide%20to%20 Section%20136%20for%20Emergency%20Departments%20-%20Dec%202017.pdf (accessed 31 May 2021).

The Royal College of Emergency Medicine (2019) *Acute Behavioural Disturbance (ABD): Guidelines on Management in Police Custody*. London: Royal College of Emergency Medicine. Available at: https://fflm.ac.uk/wp-content/uploads/2019/05/ AcuteBehaveDisturbance_Apr19-FFLM-RCEM.pdf (accessed 16 May 2021).

Urgent and Emergency Care Review programme team (2015) *Transforming Urgent and Emergency Care Services in England: Clinical Models for Ambulance Services* (guidance for commissioners regarding clinical models for ambulance services). Available at: https://www.nhs.uk/nhsengland/keogh-review/documents/uecr-ambulance-guidance-fv. pdf (accessed 30 May 2021).

World Health Organization (WHO) (2018) *International Classification of Diseases for Mortality and Morbidity Statistics* (11th revision). Available at: https://icd.who.int/ browse11/l-m/en (accessed 16 May 2021).

7 Negotiation and de-escalation

Yuet Wah Patrick

Learning objectives

- To develop a basic awareness of how to negotiate a change in another person's behaviour or thoughts
- To explore the essential components of effective communication
- To recognize signs of escalation and highlight techniques to de-escalate a situation

---

Introduction

In recent years there has been an increased awareness of violence against ambulance staff as the number of assaults against healthcare workers and emergency services staff have become a national concern. In 2019, 34 per cent of ambulance workers reported to have experienced some kind of violence at least once (NHS staff survey 2019). It is noted that in the majority of incidences that involved some kind of aggression, alcohol and/or drug consumption were a contributing factor (Institute of Alcohol Studies 2015) and the Government has recognized alcohol and substance misuse as two of the six 'main drivers of violent crimes'. In addition, alcohol and substance misuse has also been found to be a consistent predictor of aggression in people experiencing a mental health crisis (Swartz et al. 1998).

People experiencing a mental health crisis can display impetuous, unpredictable, inappropriate and irrational behaviour depending on their condition and the intensity of their crisis. Mental health is likely to play a role in a proportion of the crisis incidents that negotiators are involved with (Grubb 2010). Using alcohol or drugs as a crutch exacerbates any erratic behaviour, increasing the instability of an already volatile situation. The conflict is further intensified if the demands or wishes of the person in crisis are not met, either because they are inappropriate or unobtainable at that time. The paramedic can potentially find themselves in the difficult situation of trying to help someone in crisis who is emotionally charged, frustrated and desperate.

The power of communication, negotiation and de-escalation should not be underestimated, and indeed one may be surprised at how effective a few simple techniques can be when trying to elicit a desirable response and behaviour. A familiarization with fundamental negotiation and de-escalation strategies is crucial in preventing, or at least minimizing, aggressive behaviour. In this chapter, models of negotiation and de-escalation will be discussed with the understanding that employing certain strategies will be beneficial in dealing with the potentially aggressive encounter. It is important to note that after reading this chapter the reader will not be a trained negotiator, and attempts should not be made to deal with high-risk incidents (such as someone threatening to jump off a bridge). These situations must be left to a trained professional to resolve.

Negotiation

'Negotiation is a basic means of getting what you want from others. It is back-and-forth communication designed to reach an agreement when you and the other side have some interests that are shared and others that are opposed' (Fisher and Ury 2012).

Negotiation is needed when individuals have different goals but need to reach an agreement. For example, the goal of the person in crisis could be to hurt themselves, and the paramedic's goal is to prevent them from taking this action. Both parties need to reach an agreement that is acceptable to both sides. Successful negotiation, where an agreement is reached that both parties are willing to accept, depends on a number of factors, including identifying individual positions or standpoints; attempting to understand the other person's perspective (in this case the paramedic shows empathy as they attempt to understand why the person wants to hurt themselves); and gaining their trust to promote a change in their behaviour (Van Hasselt et al. 2008).

The fundamental goal of negotiation is to change an individual's behaviour or actions. In a crisis or emergency situation, the paramedic should guide the person in distress through progressive stages of negotiation, supporting them throughout the process until the person is willing to make that change. In order to do this, an understanding of the change process and how to effectively influence someone's mindset is therefore central to a positive outcome (Gredecki 2011).

Position vs interest

Conflict arises when there is a disparity between the positions or opinions of two or more people. In brief, it is when two or more people do not agree on something. The beginnings of any resolution can only be brought about if the position of each individual is made clear, providing an anchor from which discussions can begin (Fisher and Ury 2012). Interestingly, often the individuals involved have similar interests but differing positions. For example, the individual who is at crisis point and has resorted to taking extreme action such as suicide ideation wants to find a solution to stop them feeling the way they are, and the only option they can see at that time is through suicide. The paramedic also wants to find a solution to stop the cause of the other person's crisis, and hence shares the same interest, but their position is to preserve life, not end it. Thus, a conflict in positions is created.

Once a conflict in positions is determined, the paramedic must work to facilitate a change in the other person's position while resisting becoming fixated on their own position and 'winning'. Adopting a 'winning' approach risks locking the other person into their current position as they are afraid of 'losing face' by backing down and 'losing' the negotiation (Fisher and Ury 2012). The key is for the paramedic to explore the reasons for the difference in positions and facilitate the change process by giving the person in crisis a sense of autonomy in bringing about the change – i.e. making the other person think it is their idea to change their behaviour because they think it is a better option. Motivating a change in the individual's mindset can be very challenging, and requires an understanding of the negotiation process and skill in its execution.

The stages of negotiation

Individuals experiencing a mental health crisis often display self-destructive behaviour motivated by anger, frustration or depression (St Yves and Veyrat 2012). Their reactions can be unpredictable and/or inappropriate due to the anxiety and stress that they are feeling. Three core skills – active listening and communication, empathy and building a rapport – are instrumental to successful negotiation and de-escalation, and will be revisited throughout this chapter.

Crisis intervention in negotiation encompasses four primary stages: (1) dealing with emotions, (2) establishing communication, (3) identifying the precipitating event(s), and (4) problem solving.

Dealing with emotions – expressing empathy

A person's behaviour is strongly influenced by the emotions that person holds about their experience. It is these emotions that create the crisis situation rather than the event itself. For example, an isolated event of losing a job or ending a relationship is unlikely to push a person to crisis point, but the emotions of stress, anxiety, frustration, guilt, hurt or anger could do. Acknowledgement of and addressing these emotions is key to influencing behaviour and motivating change (Vecchi et al. 2005).

In addressing emotions, it is important not to make assumptions about how the person is feeling. For example, a paramedic who attempts to be empathetic and says 'I know how you feel' could be counterproductive as the person either does not believe them, or is upset because the paramedic is devaluing their experience by talking about themselves and has therefore changed the focus of the conversation away from their own perspective. An alternative, 'I can't imagine what you are going through but I would like to try to understand, if you could explain to me how you are feeling', tells the person in crisis that the paramedic is trying to understand their position while offering them the opportunity to express their feelings, thus validating their reality (Noesner and Webster 1997).

Empathy

An understanding of what the other person is thinking and what their perspective is on the situation allows the paramedic to identify the disparity between their own views and the views of the other person, giving a starting point on how to reduce the amount of conflict. For example, if the paramedic finds out the reason why the individual is refusing help or treatment is because of previous bad experiences, the paramedic can work with that and find out what the individual did not like about their experience and offer alternatives that may be more satisfactory.

It is important to note that it is not the person's thoughts or feelings that are the problem in a crisis situation, it is their behaviour that is the issue. Telling the person that their thoughts and feelings are understandable due to their experiences promotes comprehension and trust between the two parties, making the individual feel that they are not alone and that someone is on their side. Explaining that it is their behaviour or actions that are the problem will help them see that there are alternative ways to deal with their situation, and that now they have someone to support them, they can change their behaviour.

A person experiencing delusions or hallucinations can be particularly difficult to deal with as their delusions and hallucinations are very real to them, making their actions unpredictable and challenging. Care should be taken to avoid collusion with any delusions, but questions should be asked about them to give insight into the person's world, allowing the paramedic to validate their experience and make sense of their situation (Hart 2014).

Once different viewpoints have been identified and empathy is initiated, the paramedic can attempt to build a rapport. Without empathy, an effective rapport cannot be established.

Establishing communication (rapport building/active listening)

The impact of effective communication techniques has been well versed in healthcare. A combination of regard to body language, tone and intonation of voice, employing active listening techniques and being non-judgemental contribute to being able to communicate effectively.

Tone, intonation and body language are important to check as these elements speak louder than the actual words spoken. Being non-judgemental is crucial, as a person in crisis often judges themselves harshly and negatively through the eyes of others. The paramedic needs to work extra hard to maintain a neutral view that will not upset the other person.

Active listening

Active listening enables the listener to hear and understand other people's thoughts and experience the conversation through their lens, instead of forcing their own thoughts immediately into the situation. It allows the speaker to be heard, which is often all they want. Advice can be given at a later time, when the person is ready to receive it, if that time comes at all.

Studies have shown that most people are poor or inefficient listeners due to a variety of reasons. It is not a skill that is generally taught, unlike reading, writing or speaking, despite the fact that on average 45 per cent of a person's time is spent listening, as opposed to 30 per cent of time spent speaking in a day (Adler et al. 2017). Another reason why people are poor listeners is that, on average, a person has the capacity to understand 400 spoken words per minute but to speak at a rate of 125 words per minute. This disparity in rates means that only 25 per cent of brain capacity is being used when listening, which allows scope for minds to wander as the brain is looking for something to do (Adler et al. 2017).

Bad listening habits need to be replaced by good listening habits for active listening to take place. Before looking at recognized active listening techniques, it is useful to identify some bad habits that need to be eliminated.

Overexposure – a paramedic may have heard the same story over and over again during the span of their career and can risk becoming robotic in their approach. Showing a lack of interest or impatience as the paramedic waits for the person to finish their story should absolutely be avoided. Focusing on really listening to what the person is saying will provide insight on how the paramedic can help to resolve the situation. The person in crisis will pick up on 'wasting someone's time' and being a 'burden', so it is important to show an interest and engage in what they are saying.

Interrupting the speaker, or jumping in to say something when the speaker pauses as they think of what they are going to say next, drastically reduces listening efficiency, resulting in the speaker not being heard. If the speaker makes a statement that the paramedic disagrees with, the paramedic must let the other person finish what they are saying in order to try to understand how they are in the position they find themselves in. People have a difference of opinions as a result of different beliefs, cultures, upbringing and experiences. Statements may be made that the paramedic disagrees with, which could make them angry or upset, but it is essential they remain impartial to the conversation.

Intense concentration is needed on the listener's behalf when actively listening. Some simple active listening techniques can be adopted to enhance the communication between the paramedic and the person in need.

Mirroring and paraphrasing show the speaker that the listener is attentive, keeping the focus on the person in distress rather than on the listener. Mirroring involves repeating what the person in crisis has said almost verbatim, whereas paraphrasing repeats what the listener has heard and understood in their own words.

Through mirroring and paraphrasing, the speakers hear how they express themselves to others, allowing them insight into how they may feel and how others may perceive their situation. They also allow the listener to confirm if they have heard correctly, and in the case of paraphrasing, whether they have understood what they are being told.

Affect labelling identifies a person's emotions by putting them into words. Naming emotions allows the individual to put 'distance' between themselves and their emotions, thus detaching themselves from the situation (Torre and Lieberman 2018). Affect labelling gives the individual the opportunity to reflect on how they are feeling and make sense of their emotions. For example, if the paramedic says *'You sound angry'* or *'You seem upset'* the individual can confirm if the right emotion has been interpreted and what sense they make of it.

Summarizing involves taking the key points of what the listener has heard and reiterating them in a logical and clear way. It allows clarification for both parties; the paramedic can check that they have heard and interpreted what the speaker has said correctly, and the speaker has the opportunity to correct any misunderstandings.

An example of summarizing might be: *'I want to check that I understand what you're saying; your partner hasn't responded to your phone calls for no apparent reason [paraphrase] and this makes you angry [affect labelling].'*

Open-ended questioning allows the individual to explore their emotions with the aim of decreasing their emotional state, bringing them down to a level that allows for more rational thinking. Open-ended questions typically start with *'What'* or *'When'* or statements such as *'Tell me more about that'*. *'Why'* statements are usually avoided, as they tend to be perceived as interrogatory.

Effective pauses are deliberate pauses where listeners can harness the power of silence for effect at appropriate times. People often feel uncomfortable with silence and seek to jump in to fill spaces in a conversation to avoid feeling awkward. If the listener consistently fills the silence by talking then this may discourage the individual from speaking, and in some cases the roles of the speaker and listener may be reversed. In addition, an agitated person can often be calmed with silence as it is difficult for them to maintain their emotions if there is no one to add fuel to the fire.

Minimal encouragers are short, well-timed verbal responses such as *'yes'*, *'go on'*, *'I see' and 'okay'*, which effectively tell the speaker that the listener is attentive and encourage them to continue talking.

'I' statements are used by the listener when they feel it is appropriate to make a personal observation to further develop rapport. This is useful to connect an emotion or experience that the speaker is describing. For example, the paramedic may say, *'I am concerned that we haven't come to an agreement yet. What else do you think we can do to help this situation?'* This statement tells the individual that the paramedic cares that a suitable solution has not been found, and also offers collaboration and autonomy to the distressed person as they are asked for their suggestions.

There is no set pattern or structure when active listening. Practising and employing active listening techniques will help the paramedic improve their skills, however a combination of communication techniques and genuineness is essential to avoid the paramedic from coming across as robotic or scripted. Genuineness is important to build rapport (Hart 2014).

Rapport

Rapport is the creation of a trusting relationship and is essential in motivating change in behaviour. Active listening and being empathetic are instrumental in building rapport, and if these stages are executed well then there is a greater chance of creating a good rapport. Simple tactics can be employed in developing rapport and trust, such as looking for common ground; being courteous and respectful to each other; being interested and attentive to each other; being honest and giving truthful responses (while being diplomatic); and finally, being genuine.

If the individual is resistant in working with the paramedic, the paramedic should not challenge them, but should instead provide opportunities for the individual to question why they do not want to accept suggestions being made. For example, if the paramedic is told to *'just leave me alone, I don't want your help'*, it is helpful to find out why the other person is refusing help by asking *'can you tell me why you don't want any help from me?'* rather than challenging them by saying *'well, I can't leave you like this so we need to work something out'*.

The paramedic should take this opportunity to reflect on their own thoughts or behaviour to see if there are any attributes that may have influenced the person's reluctance to work with them. For example, the paramedic may have:

- a lack of insight into the person's mental state or view of the world
- minimized the problem or not validated the situation
- a desire to maintain control of the situation, therefore failing to give the individual autonomy
- differing views and beliefs to the person
- carried residue or distracting emotions with them from a previous incident or from outside work

Once the paramedic has checked their own biases they can go on to examine their questioning style:

- Does the person understand the question?
- Could the question be phrased in a more understandable way?
- Does the person feel too embarrassed to answer?
- Is the question too distressing or threatening to answer at this time?
- Was it the 'right' question for that stage of the interview? (Hart 2014)

People in distress are likely to be experiencing some degree of anxiety, if not directly as a consequence of their mental state then in relation to being 'assessed', which they may equate with being 'judged' or having possible negative outcomes. To minimize their distress, the paramedic must adopt a calm approach, actively listen to the distressed person's concerns, be non-judgemental in their responses and actions, and set boundaries if required (Hart 2014).

Identifying the precipitating event(s)

The precipitating event is often a significant loss (e.g. spouse, job, money) which is the 'last straw' or 'trigger' that propels a person into crisis (Vecchi et al. 2005). Due to high levels of emotion, the person in crisis is often confused about the impact of the precipitating event, resulting in inappropriate actions. The precipitating events are the 'hooks' which must be focused on to resolve the crisis (Vecchi et al. 2005). For example, a man has severely harmed himself after his wife told him that she was leaving him with their children. The 'hook' is the anticipated loss (of the children and the relationship). By providing justification for this behaviour (e.g. *'You are feeling hurt as you have lost someone and people you love have been taken away from you, which is why you are hurting yourself. But you can still enjoy a relationship with your children once you stop hurting yourself and you can look after them'*), the actions of the estranged husband are positively reframed. This serves to alleviate internal conflict, defuse negative emotions and set the stage for subsequent problem solving and crisis resolution.

Problem solving

Once emotions are better controlled, communication has been established and the triggering event has been identified and discussed, the individual is more likely to be receptive to problem solving. This stage involves looking at possible solutions that are acceptable to both the person in crisis and the paramedic. Throughout the process, unacceptable options are eliminated while the benefits and downfalls of acceptable solutions are explored, until the most appropriate one is selected. As the individual is engaged in the process, they are more willing to change their behaviour as they can see it is a suitable option (Gredecki 2011).

A person in crisis will find problem solving extremely difficult and will need to be guided through the process of how to do this (Hart 2014).

The following theories have been developed or adopted by police negotiators in hostage situations. Nevertheless, certain principles from these theories can be applied to the crisis situation with a mentally disturbed person.

Principled negotiation (win–win model)

The win–win model seeks to effectively improve (or at least not damage) the relationship between the two parties, addressing four principles:

- *Separate the people from the problem* – this principle identifies the behaviour as the problem, not the person, and involves building a rapport with the person to help find a solution to the problem.
- *Focus on interests, not positions* – finding out what the other person's needs are (there is usually more than one need) is the focus here rather than the positions the individual and the paramedic have found themselves in. Once the person's needs have been established, then they can work with the paramedic to look at solutions.
- *Create options for mutual gain* – brainstorming a range of options and choosing ones that are acceptable to both parties is the emphasis of this principle.
- *Insist on using objective criteria* – this entails deciding on solutions that allow both parties to feel they have achieved something, rather than one party 'winning' and the other one 'losing'.

This model supports the notion that conflict arises when two people hold opposing positions. Adopting an empathetic approach allows the paramedic to understand the other person's perspective and the emotions that underpin it. It is also important for the paramedic to review and understand their own position, as influencing factors may also create a barrier to a successful outcome. For example, the paramedic may not have any children, and therefore may struggle to relate to the loss that the estranged husband in the earlier example feels. This may initially make them think that the person is overreacting and acting irrationally. However, acknowledging this lack of connection may be enough to make the paramedic think and review their position before proceeding. If the distressed person feels that their point of view is being listened to, then they are more likely to entertain alternative options suggested.

Structured Tactical Engagement Process (STEPS)

The STEPS model views the crisis situation as a behavioural problem in which change must be brought about (Kelln and McMurtry 2007). It is based on Prochaska and DiClemente's transtheoretical stages of change model (1982), which was developed to modify behaviours to achieve goals such as losing weight or quitting smoking.

The STEPS model consists of four steps, starting with the person in crisis becoming aware of the situation (Step 0) and ending with voluntary surrender (Step 3).

Step 0: Precontemplation stage – the individual is unwilling to acknowledge that the situation or their behaviour needs to change and is therefore
uncooperative in their actions. The focus at this stage is to build a rapport
and make a connection with the individual to enable progression to the
next step. In this first stage individuals may make unrealistic requests or
simply demand that the police or ambulance crew leave the premises.

Step 1: Contemplation stage – the individual realizes that their behaviour
must change if the situation is to be resolved, but they are not quite sure
how to go about implementing this as they do not have the resources or
confidence to do so. At this stage, encouragement and reassurance should
be offered to increase the individual's confidence, creating hope.

Step 2: Preparation stage – the individual has identified that there is a
problem and that their behaviour needs to change. They may explore
various possibilities (such as agreeing to treatment or transport to hospital). The paramedic's role becomes more proactive and directive as they
explore options to develop an appropriate exit strategy that will maintain
dignity and save face.

Step 3: Action – the individual carries out the agreed plan. The paramedic
remains supportive and directive throughout, until the action has been
completed.

The Behavioural Influencing Stairway Model

The Behavioural Influencing Stairway Model (BISM) (Vecchi 2007) is an
updated version of the Behavioural Change Stairway Model (BCSM) devised
by the FBI's Crisis Negotiation Unit. It consists of five stages: 1) active listening

Figure 7.1 The Behavioural Influence Stairway Model (BISM)

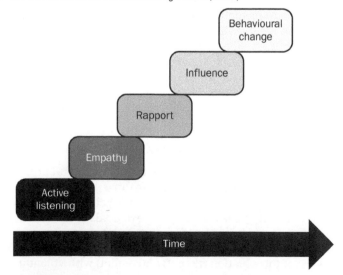

Adapted from the BISM (Vecchi 2007)

skills, 2) empathy, 3) rapport, 4) influence and 5) behavioural change, progressing from getting the person to engage to motivating change in behaviour.

The BISM process is sequential and cumulative in that the stages must be taken in order and each stage must be achieved or completed before progressing to the next stage. This means that stage 1, active listening, must be accomplished before progressing to stage 2, empathy, and so on. However, the BISM does state that active listening should continue through each stage, as it recognizes that the success of each stage depends on implementing this skill.

Active listening

People in crisis want to be heard and understood. Active listening attends to this need and is critical for developing a relationship that will ultimately lead to behavioural change and crisis resolution (Noesner and Webster 1997).

Empathy

Empathy is a natural by-product of effective active listening. It enables the paramedic to try to understand the situation through the eyes of the person in crisis. The goal is to establish a position whereby a rapport can be developed.

Rapport

Up to this stage of the BISM, the relationship has been one-sided; the person in crisis has been talking and the paramedic has been actively listening and empathetic. As empathy is shown, rapport develops, which increases trust and mutual affinity. Once a rapport has been developed, the person in crisis begins coming to terms with what has happened and is more likely to listen to (and accept) what the paramedic has to offer. At this stage, the paramedic and the distressed person begin to explore 'face saving' justifications which are more successful in getting the individual to agree with any proposals (Browning et al. 2011). This involves offering reasons to justify any unacceptable behaviour, providing a lifeline the individual can grasp to get themselves out of the situation they have created without losing face.

Influence

At this stage, a relationship has been established and the individual is willing to work with the paramedic to find solutions to the situation that are acceptable to both parties. The paramedic has earned the trust of the individual to instigate behaviour change.

Behavioural change

As mentioned earlier, if the previous four stages have been successfully completed then there is a higher chance that behavioural change will occur, as a positive relationship has developed between the two parties. Agreed actions are implemented without conflict. Obstacles to reaching this final stage include the negotiator omitting stages or moving too rapidly through the stages (Vecchi et al. 2005).

SCARF

Rock (2008) created the 'SCARF' model, which is based on neuroscience and denotes that the brain promotes certain behaviours to minimize threats and maximize rewards. The brain is constantly looking out for stimuli that may lead to a threat or a reward, and sends signals to the body to act accordingly. Brain activity in a reward state, which is detected as a positive emotion, is stimulated in the frontal lobe, which is responsible for abstract thinking, self-management and problem solving. The brain analyses the situation and signals are sent out to say that it is safe to engage. A person experiencing a negative emotion, and in a threatened state, shows more brain activity in the limbic system, where the amygdala (fight or flight) takes over. In this case, rational thinking and reasoning are limited as the person goes towards fight or flight mode.

The SCARF model classifies five domains – status, certainty, autonomy, relatedness and fairness – which can be used to avoid triggering threatening responses and encourage rewarding responses.

Status is one's sense of importance or worth in relation to others. Threat is perceived if the individual feels that their rank or status is challenged, and it is rewarded when the person feels valued. It is interesting to note here that the presence of uniformed professionals, such as paramedics and the police, can trigger either the reward or the threat response in this domain depending on how the person in crisis feels about themselves. By showing empathy and actively listening, the paramedic attempts to stimulate the reward response, making the individual more receptive to engaging in finding a solution to the situation.

Certainty refers to the familiarity and recognition of a situation. Uncertain or new experiences increase stress levels, which is a threat response, decreasing the brain's capacity to process what is going on. The use of clear and simple language to explain any expectations or goals to the person is instrumental at this stage as their brain struggles to process any complex information or thoughts.

Autonomy is the sense of control a person feels they have over a situation. More control equals a higher reward response; less control equals a higher threat response. Giving the individual choices promotes their autonomy and thus their engagement.

Relatedness refers to a sense of belonging or acceptance. Reward responses are triggered by empathy and rapport building in this domain as the individual is made to feel that they are valued and understood. Taking time to develop this domain is worthwhile as it is instrumental in gaining the trust and cooperation of the individual.

Fairness is a lack of favouritism to one side or the other. It is the basis of compromise as both parties strive to get what they want. If the person in distress feels that they are being ignored or treated unfairly, a threat response is triggered, making them upset or angry. However, if they sense they are being treated fairly, their reward system produces a sense of satisfaction.

De-escalation

The key to preventing escalation is to instigate negotiation early on, and if negotiation is not appropriate or is failing, recognition of the precursors to aggression is essential to warn the paramedic to change tack and employ de-escalation techniques. However, negotiation or early identification of escalation is not always possible, especially in the pre-hospital environment due to the situation already escalating or reaching its peak of emotion prior to the arrival of the paramedic on the scene. If the situation intensifies to aggression or the paramedic has arrived at the height of escalation, then de-escalation techniques must be adopted to defuse the situation for the safety of the individual and everyone present, including the paramedic themselves.

The rest of this chapter will look at how to recognize the signs of the agitated person as the situation escalates and techniques that can be employed to defuse a situation.

What is de-escalation and when should it be used?

De-escalation is a psychosocial intervention, which should be used as a first-line response to aggression and violence (NICE 2015) as it is the least restrictive method when managing a potentially violent situation. De-escalation comprises a set of skills, knowledge and personal qualities in the domains of communication, self-regulation, assessment, activity and safety maintenance with the aim of reducing or eliminating aggression (Hallett 2018).

While negotiation facilitates the communication between two parties with the end goal of reaching a mutually satisfactory result/outcome, de-escalation involves defusing a volatile situation where negotiation is not appropriate, either because the person was already in a heightened state before the paramedic arrived and needs to be calmed before discussions can start, or because attempts at negotiation have failed.

Once the aggression has subsided, negotiation may commence or continue, if appropriate.

Causes of escalation/aggression

Numerous factors on both the aggressor's and the paramedic's behalf can contribute to a situation escalating to aggression:

- The paramedic engages in a power struggle and wants to 'win' the argument
- The paramedic does not observe the person's body language and identify precursors to escalation
- The paramedic becomes emotionally involved and overreacts to threats and abuse
- The person in distress feels they are not being heard; they have lost their dignity, control and autonomy; they feel threatened or disempowered; their issues are minimized or undervalued (Price and Baker 2012)

Certain behaviours have been recognized as antecedents to escalation. Often, but not always, aggression is preceded by agitation. Therefore, it is logical to intercept at the point of agitation in order to prevent the situation from escalating (Lavelle et al. 2016).

Inappropriate or provoking behaviour can be antecedents to aggression – for instance rule-breaking, non-compliance, self-exposure, as well as self-harm and suicide attempts (Hallett and Dickens 2017). In the pre-hospital environment, these behaviours could be demonstrated as refusing treatment, smoking when asked not to, derogatory or challenging comments being made.

What are the signs of agitation?

Luck et al. (2007) studied the behaviour of violent patients in the emergency department and recognized that many patients displayed certain behaviours before becoming aggressive. The mnemonic STAMP was created to encompass the behaviours that they identified as precursors to escalation. Although the study took place in emergency department, the same precursors can be applied in the out-of-hospital setting.

- **S**taring is an important early indicator of potential violence used to intimidate the recipient into taking action. Addressing the issue rather than ignoring it or skirting around it often placates the individual, avoiding aggression. Lack of eye contact is also associated with anger and passive resistance. However, it is important to note that there can be cultural reasons for avoiding eye contact which should be taken into consideration.
- **T**one and volume of voice mostly involves raised voices and yelling, but can also include sarcastic and caustic replies.
- **A**nxiety is especially marked with mental health crisis and if substance abuse is involved.
- **M**umbling, using slurred or incoherent speech, repeatedly asking the same question or making the same statements may be observed in some people. Mumbling is perceived to be a sign of mounting frustration and a cue for violence.
- **P**acing is an indication of mounting agitation. Other physical indicators included staggering, waving arms around or pulling away from healthcare staff trying to treat them.

Stages of de-escalation

As with negotiation, no one strategy of de-escalation fits all. A flexible and creative approach is often needed in combination with recognized de-escalation techniques to address the needs of the individual. The methods employed rely on the intuition of the paramedic. Elements such as active listening, empathy and rapport are fundamental for effective de-escalation as they are for negotiation.

Kaplan and Wheeler (1983) identified a cycle of stages a person would experience when going through a crisis, and called this the five phases of assault. It comprises of the following stages.

Trigger

The trigger is the cause of whatever initiates the person's anger or aggression. It could be something obvious such as having an argument, or it could be something less evident that perhaps occurred hours or even days ago that the person has been dwelling on. Its significance may seem overinflated to others, but it is nonetheless important and a trigger for the individual.

In this phase, it is still possible for the person to be calmed.

Escalation

As the person's anger grows their adrenaline level increases, affecting their ability to think and act rationally. While it is less likely that the person will be able to calm themselves during this phase, it is still possible for others to intervene and prevent the individual reaching the crisis phase.

Crisis

The crisis phase occurs when the person becomes increasingly physiologically, emotionally and psychologically aroused, making it difficult for them to think or act rationally. They become abusive and threatening. De-escalation techniques are unlikely to be effective and the main focus at this stage is to ensure the safety of everyone present.

Recovery

The person becomes fatigued, and as their anger or aggression subsides they enter the recovery phase, gradually returning to their baseline mood and behaviours. However, it can take at least 90 minutes for adrenaline levels to return to normal, so although the immediate crisis may have passed, the person's anger can easily be reignited.

Post-crisis

In this phase, the person may feel remorse for what has occurred and their mood dips below their baseline mood before returning to normal.

The time frame for each stage varies from minutes to hours (with the exception of the time it takes for adrenaline levels to return to normal). In the case of rapid progression from trigger to crisis, it can be challenging to identify the trigger to the behaviour (Bowers et al. 2011).

Hallett (2018) observe a model of de-escalation comprising three tiers: primary, secondary and tertiary prevention.

Primary prevention aims to reduce the risk of challenging behaviour occurring in the first instance and corresponds closely to negotiation techniques discussed earlier in this chapter. Tactics such as removing the person from the source of emotional upset and taking them to a quieter location where their anger cannot be fuelled by others present can help at this stage.

Secondary prevention looks at the actions taken to reduce the risk of escalating behaviour in order to avoid the situation reaching crisis stage. The core elements of effective communication including active listening, empathy and rapport building are present at this stage.

Tertiary prevention focuses on minimizing the physical aggression. When there is an imminent risk of harm from violent behaviour, the purpose of intervention changes from de-escalating the situation to preserving the physical safety of those involved or present.

Throughout the de-escalation process, paramedics should constantly dynamically risk assess the situation. This means a 'continuous process of identifying hazards and risks and taking steps to eliminate or reduce them in the rapidly changing circumstances of an incident' (NHS Counter Fraud and Security Management Division 2007) should be performed, and involves paramedics:

- Being alert to warning signs
- Ensuring that they are in a position to physically remove themselves from the environment if necessary
- Judging the best course of action, for example whether to continue the interaction or withdraw
- Assessing the need for physical security measures, for example calling for assistance from other staff, security or the police

The dynamic risk assessment should begin with a 'ten-second risk assessment', whereby if the paramedic feels there is a risk of harm to themselves or others, they should immediately withdraw to a place of safety (NHS Counter Fraud and Security Management Division 2007).

The paramedic may call for assistance from other healthcare staff, security or the police to ensure safety. While additional support is often necessary, it should be noted that 'a show of force' may escalate a situation (Duperouzel 2008). Therefore, careful assessment of the situation is required.

Physical intervention may be necessary where de-escalation and other interventions have failed (NICE 2015). The risks involved with incorrect application of physical interventions include mental trauma, physical injury and possibly death, therefore physical intervention should only be employed by appropriately trained people and as a last resort (NICE 2015).

De-escalation techniques

Once an individual has reached a level of agitation or aggression, it is not possible to reason with them. Their emotions must be reduced before rational discussions can take place. Certain qualities have been recognized as desirable for effective de-escalators, as they gain the individual's trust. These include being honest, approachable, supportive, self-aware, empathetic with genuine concern, non-judgemental, confident and appearing non-threatening and non-authoritarian (Duperouzel 2008). These qualities help people develop feelings of hope, security and self-acceptance (Finfgeld-Connett 2009), paving the way for effective negotiation.

In addition to the skills already mentioned such as active listening, showing empathy and building a rapport, there are several techniques that are useful in de-escalating a situation which can be employed in the pre-hospital setting:

- Appear calm – taking several breaths before interacting with the agitated person can assist the paramedic with remaining calm, or at least giving the impression that they are calm, even if they are not. Remaining calm can lessen some of the effects of adrenaline, reducing the heightened state of the individual. Promoting calm can be instigated through a psychological phenomenon known as 'mood matching', whereby people replicate another person's emotions – so an angry person may make another person feel angry, but equally, a calm person may promote calmness in the other person (Echterhoff et al. 2009).

- Remove the trigger or the person from the environment to a calm and quiet place. The back of the ambulance is ideal if the person is outdoors, as it offers privacy and the person no longer has to 'perform' in front of an audience. This gives them the opportunity to calm down and change behaviour without losing face. A quiet place not only lessens the need to shout or speak with raised voices, which can further stimulate emotions, but it also minimizes misunderstandings as information can be misheard or raising frustrations as the person is asked constantly to repeat themselves due to not being heard above the noise.

- Adopt a low and neutral tone of voice to avoid overstimulation of the already heightened senses of the person in distress. It is difficult for the agitated person to maintain their anger if responses are calm and neutral.

- Keep facial expressions neutral. In heightened emotional states, facial expressions can be misinterpreted – for example, a smile could be seen as mockery and a stern face could be interpreted as aggressive or intimidating.

- Congruence between what is said and facial expressions should be checked.

- Body language must be relaxed and open, offering trust and respect which may be mirrored by the agitated person.

- Give at least double the usual amount of personal space. Elevated emotional state heightens the senses and what is deemed as acceptable in respect of personal space under normal circumstances may feel too close for the person in crisis, making them feel threatened even more. Leaving additional space is also safer for the paramedic as they are out of striking distance.
- Empathize with feelings but not with the behaviour. Let the aggressor know that while it is normal to feel the way they do, their behaviour is not acceptable. Offering alternatives will empower the person, giving them a sense of autonomy which enhances the progression of de-escalation.

Things to avoid

- Don't rush into the situation – take a moment to assess the scene. If it's not safe to stay then leave and wait for reinforcements to arrive.
- Don't speak loudly to try and make yourself heard as this raises the emotional level. Wait for a pause and speak quietly but firmly.
- Don't interpret the person's feelings – attempts to understand how the person is feeling can be made once the situation has de-escalated.
- Don't react – reactions are impulsive, and often occur without thinking. Responses, on the other hand, are measured and thoughtful. Taking time to consider the situation and responding rather than reacting is beneficial. It takes an awful lot of control to appear calm in a volatile environment, and by not reacting the paramedic shows that they are still in control. It is important not to make the situation personal and react to the insults and personal abuse from the other person as this will only exacerbate the situation. This does not mean that personal attacks or insults are acceptable, but they should be addressed when the person is calm and capable of rational thought. Responding to the situation rather than reacting to it is important.
- Don't use gestures or body language that could be interpreted as aggressive. This could include finger pointing, staring, putting hands on hips.
- Don't use long, complicated sentences with jargon or terminology. Adrenaline makes it difficult to process complex information so sentences should be kept short and simple.
- Don't become frustrated if the agitated person finds it difficult to focus or understand what is being said. It may be necessary to repeat sentences or find a different way of saying it.

Conclusion

The paramedic employs varying amounts of negotiation strategies on a daily basis, in non-crisis as well as in crisis situations. Given the infinite range of possible circumstances that may be encountered in a crisis situation, a flexible and intuitive approach to negotiation and de-escalation that can be adapted to suit each individual scenario is essential. It is important to remember that the paramedic is not trained to negotiate in high-risk situations such as hostage taking or suicide threats, and these cases should be dealt with by trained negotiators. Nevertheless, employment of the core skills of active listening, empathy and rapport building, in combination with the adaptation and application of negotiation and de-escalation strategies, can result in positive and beneficial outcomes to both the paramedic and the person in crisis.

References

Adler, R.B., Rosenfeld, L.B. and Proctor, R. (2017) *Interplay: The Process of Interpersonal Communication*, 14th edn. Oxford: Oxford University Press.

Bowers, L., Stewart, D., Papadopoulos, C. et al. (2011) *Inpatient Violence and Aggression: A Literature Review*. London: King's College London.

Browning, S.L., Brockman, A.M., Van Hasselt, V.B. and Vecchi, G.M. (2011) Communications, goals and techniques, in C.A. Ireland, M. Fisher and G.M. Vecchi (eds) *Conflict and Crisis Communication: Principles and Practice*. Abingdon: Routledge, pp. 53–73.

Duperouzel, H. (2008) It's ok for people to feel angry: The exemplary management of imminent aggression, *Journal of Intellectual Disabilities*, 12(4): 295–307.

Echterhoff, G., Higgins, E. and Levine, J. (2009) Shared reality: Experiencing commonality with others' inner states about the world, *Perspectives on Psychological Science*, 4(5): 496–521.

Finfgeld-Connett, D. (2009) Management of aggression among demented or brain-injured patients, *Clinical Nursing Research*, 18(3): 272–87.

Fisher, R. and Ury, W. (2012) *Getting to Yes: Negotiating an Agreement without Giving In*, 3rd edn. London: Random House Business Books.

Gredecki, N. (2011) Negotiation: principles and theoretical underpinnings, in C.A. Ireland, M. Fisher and G.M. Vecchi (eds) *Conflict and Crisis Communication: Principles and Practice*. Abingdon: Routledge, pp. 33–52.

Grubb, A. (2010) Modern day hostage (crisis) negotiation: The evolution of an art form within the policing arena, *Aggression and Violent Behaviour*, 15(5): 341–8.

Hallett, N. (2018) Preventing and managing challenging behaviour, *Nursing Standard*, 32(26): 51–62.

Hallett, N. and Dickens, G. (2017) De-escalation of aggressive behaviour in healthcare settings: Concept analysis, *International Journal of Nursing Studies*, 75: 10–20.

Hart, C. (2014) *A Pocket Guide to Risk Assessment and Management in Mental Health*. Abingdon: Routledge.

Institute of Alcohol Studies (2015) *Alcohol's Impact on the Emergency Services*. London: IAS. Available at: https://www.ias.org.uk/wp-content/uploads/2020/09/rp18102015.pdf (accessed 21 April 2021).

Kaplan, S.G. and Wheeler, E.G. (1983) Survival skills for working with potentially violent clients, *Social Casework*, 64(6): 339–46.

Kelln, B.R.C. and McMurtry, C.M. (2007) STEPS – Structured Tactical Engagement Process: A model for crisis negotiation, *Journal of Police Crisis Negotiation*, 7(2): 29–51.

Lavelle, M., Stewart, D., James, K. et al. (2016) Predictors of effective de-escalation in acute inpatient psychiatric settings, *Journal of Clinical Nursing*, 25(15–16): 2180–8.

Luck, L., Jackson, D. and Usher, K. (2007) STAMP: Components of observable behaviour that indicate potential for patient violence in emergency departments, *Journal of Advanced Nursing*, 59(1): 11–19.

National Institute for Health and Care Excellence (NICE) (2015) *Violence and Aggression: Short-Term Management in Mental Health, Health and Community Settings.* NICE guideline NG10. London: NICE.

NHS Counter Fraud and Security Management Division (2007) *Prevention and Management of Violence Where Withdrawal of Treatment is not an Option.* London: NHS Business Services Authority.

NHS staff survey (2019) *NHS Staff Survey: Results.* Available at: https://www.nhsstaff surveyresults.com/ (accessed 22 April 2021).

Noesner, G.W. and Webster, M. (1997) Crisis intervention: Using active listening skills in negotiation, *FBI Law Enforcement Bulletin*, 66: 13–19.

Price, O. and Baker, J. (2012) Key components of de-escalation techniques: A thematic synthesis, *International Journal of Mental Health Nursing*, 21(4): 310–19.

Prochaska, J.O. and DiClemente, C.C. (1982) Transtheoretical therapy: Toward a more integrative model of change, *Psychotherapy: Theory, Research and Practice*, 19(3): 276–88.

Rock, D. (2008) SCARF: A brain-based model for collaborating with and influencing others, *NeuroLeadership Journal*, 1: 1–9.

St Yves, M. and Veyrat, J.P. (2012) Negotiation models for crisis situations, in I. Collins and M. St Yves (eds) *The Psychology of Crisis Intervention for Law Enforcement Officers.* Toronto: Carswell, pp. 23–40.

Swartz, M.S., Swanson, J.W., Hiday, V.A., Borum, R., Wagner, H.R. and Burns, B.J. (1998) Violence and severe mental illness: The effects of substance abuse and nonadherence to medication, *American Journal of Psychiatry*, 155(2): 226–31.

Torre, J.B. and Lieberman, M.D. (2018) Putting feelings into words: Affect labelling as implicit emotion regulation, *Emotion Review*, 10(2): 116–24.

Van Hasselt, V.B., Romano, S.J. and Vecchi, G.M. (2008) Role playing: Applications in hostage and crisis negotiation skills training, *Behavior Modification*, 32(2): 248–63.

Vecchi, G. M. (2007). Crisis communication: Skills building in an online environment (unpublished manuscript). Behavioral Science Unit, FBI Academy, Quantico, VA. Cited in Van Hasselt, V., Romano, S. & Vecchi, G. (2008) Role playing: Applications in hostage and crisis negotiation skills training, *Behavior Modification*, 32, pp. 248–263.

Vecchi, G.M., Van Hasselt, V.B. and Romano, S. (2005) Crisis (hostage) negotiation: Current strategies and issues in high-risk conflict resolution, *Aggression and Violent Behavior*, 10(5): 533–51.

8 Suicide, breaking bad news and grief

Paula Gardner

Learning objectives

- To explore strategies when communicating bad news to family members, including models for breaking bad news
- To consider how to manage breaking bad news to children
- To explore the theories of grief and the normal stages of the grieving process
- To discuss complicated grief and the impact of death by suicide
- To highlight cultural differences to consider when dealing with death

Introduction

Caring for the loved ones of a patient who has died suddenly, unexpectedly or under traumatic circumstances can be especially challenging for paramedics. Managing bereavement is an important aspect of pre-hospital practice and it is essential that clinicians have the necessary communication skills to deliver bad news effectively, as this can play a vital part in the way a person will grieve. It is important that paramedics understand the normal grieving process and the initial needs of a person who has been informed of the death of a loved one, in order to provide effective care and support.

Ambulance staff are not expected to be bereavement specialists, but the way in which bad news is communicated, the information given and the attitude and demeanour of the crew in the initial phases following a death, are thought to have a significant impact on the recovery process. This chapter will explore how paramedics can positively influence the grieving process by effective death notification and identify how inadequate communication can have a potentially long-term adverse effect. We will also look at current models for breaking bad news that can be adapted for paramedics involved in this difficult task. Delivering bad news is stressful for paramedics, and using a structured approach and feeling prepared for the demanding task has been shown to result in improved physiological well-being for both the patient and the clinician after the news has been delivered (Walker 2018).

Breaking bad news

Breaking bad news (BBN) and managing those affected by death is quite well documented for the in-hospital environment, however out of hospital there is little research. Paramedics often feel unprepared, and this is an aspect of paramedic practice that never gets any easier.

BBN predominantly relates to out-of-hospital cardiac arrest or termination of resuscitation and subsequently delivering the notification of death to family and loved ones on scene. Bad news is termed by Narayanan et al. (2010) as information that can drastically and negatively impact a person's perception of their future. Cole (2019) highlights that the way in which bad news is communicated is just as important as the information that is given. Therefore, breaking bad news to patients in an appropriate and empathetic way is an important task which has a significant impact on the recipient.

Predominantly, research around BBN is focused on areas such as oncology, particularly around breaking the news of a cancer diagnosis to patients, but there is emerging research in obstetrics, paediatrics, trauma and general practice (Bowyer et al. 2010). There are a number of models used within hospital settings but there is currently no specific model for breaking bad news in the pre-hospital field. Park et al. (2010) acknowledge that many of the existing models are difficult to adapt to pre-hospital practice due to the unexpected nature of the environment and the challenges clinicians face with trying to create a rapport prior to delivering bad news. They do however believe that the SPIKES model could be a useful tool for BBN in the emergency setting, which will be reviewed later in this chapter.

There are inevitable anxieties which can arise due to this highly emotive aspect of the paramedic role. Iserson (2000) suggests that paramedics need to mentally prepare themselves to cope and be aware of their own anxieties and emotions which result from breaking bad news to loved ones. It is important to recognize the potential need for emotional support and well-being for paramedics in their unpredictable role – it is impossible to emotionally prepare for what may be faced during a shift. One thing they can be prepared for is the likelihood that, at some point during the day, they may need to break bad news (Maunder and Maguire 2017). With stress being identified as a leading cause of ill health among ambulance service personnel, ambulance services are recognizing that there is a growing need to support the mental health of their workforce, and many trusts are offering opportunities for health promotion aimed at reducing sickness levels. Although stress is a factor in the majority of ill health, there are no clear links to any one aspect of the paramedic role. The mental health charity MIND launched the Blue Light Programme in 2015 following an online survey which indicated that 87 per cent of emergency staff and volunteers reported having experienced poor mental health at some point in their career (MIND 2016). In 2019, a review showed that the proportion of personnel who said they were aware of mental health support available to them had risen from 46 per cent in 2015 to 65 per cent, and a significant increase was seen in respondents who said their organizations encouraged them to talk about mental health – from 29 per cent to 64 per cent. Figures also suggested that organizations are improving mental health support, with figures growing from 34 per cent to 53 per cent.

Breaking bad news in the pre-hospital environment presents many challenges, including the environment in which the news is being delivered, limited time available to spend with the bereaved and the fact there is not a traditional clinician–patient relationship. These factors can heighten the stress for both clinician and recipient, which can increase the risk of complicating the grieving process. In a study conducted on emergency department physicians' experiences with BBN, many reported finding the responses of family members such as anger or hysteria particularly difficult to deal with (Shoenberger et al. 2013).

Effective communication skills are important for all aspects of the paramedic role, and when breaking bad news these skills are key to ensuring an effective, empathetic and sensitive approach. Verbal and non-verbal communication, including active listening, is essential. Using a BBN model can help to provide structure and focus when faced with the difficult task of delivering devastating news.

SPIKES model

One of the most well-known BBN frameworks is the six-step SPIKES model, which stands for: Setting, Perception, Invitation, Knowledge, Emotions, Strategy and summary.

Setting – One of the difficulties for paramedics, often beyond their control, is the setting or environment in which the bad news has to be delivered. It is important to consider this factor and to try where possible to ensure the setting is conducive for a discussion to take place. This involves avoiding members of the public, limiting noise, for instance moving to the side of the road or taking the family to a quiet room in the house, or using the back of the ambulance if in a public place.

Perception – It is important to understand the perceptions of the family – are they aware of the serious nature of the situation, has the death been expected? Assess how much they already know about the condition of the patient.

Invitation – Ask the family if they are happy for you to explain what has happened and ask for permission to provide information around the circumstances.

Knowledge – Provide information concisely, avoiding both medical jargon and euphemisms that could be misinterpreted, such as 'moved on' or 'passed on'. Ensure the family has understood what you have said and give them sufficient knowledge to understand clearly.

Allow time for questions and for the recipient to respond to the information you have given them.

Emotions – Address the emotions of the family by showing empathy and
  understanding of the impact that the bad news has had on them.
Strategy and summary – Summarize the discussion and discuss a strategy
  for the next steps. In unexpected deaths it is likely that police attendance
  may be necessary. It is important to explain this to the family and the
  reasons for police involvement. Local policies may differ, so it is important
  to follow protocols and explain these fully to the family.

While the SPIKES model is widely used in the medical field, providing a robust
structure to follow when breaking bad news to families, it has been criticized
for its linear and sequential approach. Marschollek et al. (2019) believe that this
model can impersonalize the discussion and that it disregards the importance
of interaction between the clinician and recipient. Another limitation highlighted by Tan et al. (2019) is that the model is intended for one-to-one
communication, but it is more likely that news will be delivered to more than
one person at the same time, and in this situation a 'one to many' approach
would be more effective.

MANAGED

Maunder and Maguire (2017) created a BBN model, based on SPIKES but
adapted to acknowledge the challenges of breaking bad news in the pre-
hospital environment.

M – Mentally setting up and preparing: Be mentally prepared that during
  the shift it is likely that bad news will need to be delivered in some way.
  Prepare by understanding and familiarizing yourself with local policies and
  procedures. If the Trust has an information pack for families, know where
  it is and be prepared to use it.
A – Able and confident practice: Managing the scene calmly, professionally
  and with confidence is of paramount importance. Maunder and Maguire
  (2017) state that when dealing with resuscitation efforts, the family should
  be considered and where possible given an opportunity to witness the
  resuscitation efforts, which may be of comfort to them.
**N – Notice survivor response and assess understanding of what has
  occurred:** Similar to the Emotions element of SPIKES, using active
  listening skills and observing the responses of the family can help to assess
  how well they understand the situation. Repeating appropriate terms that
  the family uses such as 'passed away' with confirmation that 'yes, they
  have passed away – they have died' may help them absorb the information
  in a way they understand.
A – Accurately and sensitively give information and knowledge:
  Showing empathy, using clear language and being honest is important. Try

to add relevant facts that may help to reassure loved ones, such as that their loved one's pain was under control, and be sensitive when discussing the circumstances.

G – Give time for survivors' response – hear their story: Allow time for loved ones to tell you their side of events. As well as gaining a history, it will show that you are interested and care about what they have to say.

E – Attend to survivors' Emotions and signpost to support before Exiting the scene: Ensure there is support in place for loved ones before leaving scene. This could be friends, neighbours or other family members. Allow privacy and fully explain the next steps according to local policy.

D – Debrief: Where possible, debrief with colleagues involved in the incident and talk through the events. Debriefing is an extremely important process in dealing with critical incidents, providing an opportunity to reflect upon the events and receive emotional support if required.

COMFORT

The COMFORT model is increasingly used in healthcare settings and has been deemed a less rigid and more interactive method of breaking bad news. The COMFORT stages are:

Communication – As highlighted by all models of BBN, communication should be effective, clear and concise, and adaptive to the recipients' needs by using language that is familiar to them. The use of open and closed questions and repetition allows discussions to develop naturally and is a less linear approach than the SPIKES model.

Orientation – Orientation allows the clinician to guide the family on the next steps and decisions that may need to be made for their loved one.

Mindfulness – The Mindfulness element invites clinicians to develop empathetic 'attunement' to understand and engage with other's emotions through person-centred interactions.

Family – It is believed that connecting with the family using an empathetic and emotional approach enhances the interaction (Villagran et al. 2010). Family should be involved in treatment decisions where possible; this is an aspect of the COMFORT model which is more appropriate when breaking news to a patient of a terminal illness in a hospital setting.

Ongoing – Advice on where to receive ongoing support should be given to loved ones, in accordance with local guidelines.

Reiterative – The Reiterative phase highlights the importance of using repetition to make sure the recipients have understood the information you have imparted, and is used in hospital settings to assess the patient's and family members' levels of understanding about a condition or prognosis.

Team – In hospital situations there is likely to be a team involved in the care and ongoing support of patients. In the out-of-hospital setting, a 'team' may refer to clinicians called as backup, other emergency services or referral to primary care services.

While the COMFORT model is a structured and simple model, Villagran et al. (2010) believe it is best suited for use in educating clinicians in the process of breaking bad news.

ABCDE

The ABCDE model – a simple mnemonic familiar to paramedics in approaches to clinical assessment – is another example of a structured approach to breaking bad news.

A – advanced preparation, information gathering and preparing the environment

B – build a rapport with the recipient

C – communicate effectively using clear language and good verbal and non-verbal skills

D – deal with patient and family reactions, allowing time to process emotional responses

E – show empathy: encourage and validate emotions; take time to answer questions and be aware that individual reactions will vary.

Liddicoat (2018) believes this method is intentionally broad and non-prescriptive and can be a useful tool in creating effective dialogue and a basis on which to plan how to deliver bad news effectively.

GRIEV-ING

Hobgood et al. (2013) conducted a study which concluded that the GRIEV-ING model for use in training Emergency Medical Service (EMS) personnel to break bad news helped to increase confidence and competence when breaking bad news in a simulated practice environment. The eight-stage process consists of:

G – **Gather** family members, loved ones and ensure all of them are present before continuing on to the next steps

R – **Resources**: Request additional support if available, friends, information on support services

I – **Identify**: Introduce yourself, identify the deceased by name, identify the level of knowledge and understanding of the family around the events that have occurred

E – **Educate**: Inform the family of the details of the events that have occurred and educate them on the current situation with their friend or relative

V – **Verify**: Use clear language such as 'died' to avoid misinterpretation and allow time for the information to be processed and absorbed

– Allow the loved ones time to process the information you have given them and space to deal with their emotions before continuing on to the next phase

I – **Inquire**: Answer any questions to the best of your ability

N – Nuts and bolts: Next steps such as funeral services, discuss local procedures

G – Give advice on who to contact for support, or in hospital settings this may be the department contact details for any questions which may arise later

PEWTER

Keefe-Cooperman and Brady-Amoon (2013) developed the six-step model 'PEWTER' for emergency mental health practitioners, aimed at helping them communicate with patients to develop a rapport and devise treatment strategies. The model has been used in counselling victims of crime in hospital settings and in police departments for notifying homicide victims of the death of a loved one. PEWTER is a structured method intended to aid in the difficult process of delivering bad news (Keefe-Cooperman and Brady-Amoon 2013).

Prepare – to deliver the news, prepare the recipient for receiving the news and prepare the setting so it is free from distractions

Evaluate – as in the previous models, it is important to assess what the person already knows about the incident

Warning – provide an indication of what you are going to say and allow time for the recipient to prepare, before going on to deliver the news

Telling – tell the family the news in a calm, clear and empathetic way using the 'chunking' method of giving information in stages and checking for responses afterwards so as not to overwhelm the recipient

Emotional response – observe the responses of the recipient, while being aware of your own non-verbal communication and body language

Regrouping – summarize and discuss next steps, considering individual needs and wishes

Breaking bad news to children

Communicating with children can be challenging in any situation, and when delivering bad news to children there are some important points to consider. Depending on the age of the child, they may not have developed the social skills and understanding required to process traumatic events and will require more support (Isokääntä et al. 2019). When informing a child of the death of a loved one it is vital to use age-appropriate language and answer any questions honestly. Preschool children can understand very basic explanations and information should be kept minimal and delivered in simple terms. Children of this age need to be reassured that they will be taken care of.

Adolescents have a more complex understanding of traumatic situations and information should be more detailed. Adolescents like to be involved in decision-making. Some may wish to have as much information as possible about the situation, while others may want to avoid discussion due to fear of the situation (Isokääntä et al. 2019).

For children to adjust to the death of a loved one, particularly if it is a caregiver, they need to have a realistic and coherent understanding of what has happened. Effective communication will help to reassure children that someone will still take care of their physical and emotional needs (Mitchell et al. 2006).

Breaking bad news to people with learning disabilities

People with learning disabilities will have their own opinions about being told about bad news and how they want to receive it. It is thought that healthcare professionals are underconfident when breaking bad news to people with learning disabilities, while carers often feel they want to protect them from the bad news. Giving information in small 'chunks' may help them to make sense of it. It is important to take into account the capacity and understanding of the person, considering the Mental Capacity Act. Where possible, involving the person's family, friends or carers can help them receive the support they need (Tuffrey-Wijne and Rose 2017).

Key points

- Breaking bad news effectively is an important skill for every clinician to develop
- Prepare for the discussion by gaining an understanding of the situation and consider a plan such as using a BBN model to consider the important aspects of BBN
- There is no one right way to communicate bad news, but structure can be effective when holding difficult conversations
- It is important to be accurate and empathetic, while observing emotional responses and the level of understanding of the person/people you are delivering bad news to
- Allow time for the information to be processed and avoid 'filling silences'
- Recipients of bad news will respond better to patient-centred communication
- Finish the conversation with a clear plan for the next steps (Liddicoat 2018)

Viewing of the body

There is increasing evidence surrounding the importance of the bereaved viewing the body of their loved one after death and it may be particularly important in sudden and unexpected death, especially if the bereaved was not present at the time their loved one died (Mowll 2007).

It might be considered by some healthcare practitioners that viewing the body of a loved person who has died a traumatic death could be harmful. Reny et al. (2020) believe that this is not often the case and that many suffering from the sudden loss of a loved one are grateful for the opportunity to say goodbye to the person they love. Preparing the bereaved for the experience is important, particularly if the deceased has suffered significant injuries. This could mean discussing the appearance or describing the injuries, to reduce the possibility of being shocked by the way the deceased now looks. Options such as partial or fully covered viewing could also be considered. Relatives bereaved through sudden or traumatic deaths, who opted to view the body, rarely reported any regret about doing so. It is suggested that allowing the presence of family members during emergency care can be beneficial in coming to terms with the situation, and viewing the body of their loved one helps to solidify the reality of loss, reducing the potential for complicated grief to develop (Reny et al. 2020).

Theories of grief and stages of bereavement

Dealing with death is an inevitable part of the paramedic role and it is important to understand the reactions that can be displayed by a person during the initial stages of grief.

Grief is a natural response to the loss of a loved one and the term is often used alongside 'mourning' and 'bereavement', but they all hold very different meanings. Grief is an individual response to death and can affect a person emotionally, physically, behaviourally and spiritually. Mourning is the 'outward and active expression of that grief' and is the process through which grief is dealt with (Buglass 2010). Bereavement is the phase in which grief and mourning will occur and can be a form of depression which is overcome in time.

Bowlby's (1973) theory of attachment highlights the importance of human attachments and relationships, which begin to form in early childhood. Bowlby suggested that when important bonds are threatened, significant attachment behaviours can arise such as distress, anger and protest. When the attachment is permanently lost or broken, normal biological processes can become dysfunctional, with the bereaved person experiencing the activation of attachment behaviour and the reality of the loved one's absence. Based on this theory, Bowlby believed grief evolves through a series of four intertwining stages of shock, yearning and protest, despair, and recovery.

There are several theories and models of grief, many of which share common themes.

Kubler-Ross DABDA model

A widely used model of grief was developed by Kubler-Ross in 1969 and is commonly used today in healthcare education. The five systematic stages that the bereaved were thought to pass through are:

- denial
- anger

- bargaining
- depression
- acceptance

The phases are passed through sequentially and it was thought that the time spent at each stage can vary depending on the person's individual response to grief. Although this model has influenced the understanding of grief, it has been widely criticized for being too linear. One view is that grief varies between individuals, and those who do not pass through each stage or who return to an earlier stage in the process are perceived as not experiencing the 'normal' grieving process. Buglass (2010) argues that the stage models of grief do not capture the complex, varied and unique psychological and spiritual needs of a person who is grieving, and can lead to failing to address individual needs and foster a lack of empathy.

Worden (2018) suggests that grieving should be considered as an active process that involves working through four tasks:

1 **To accept the reality of the loss** – The first task in the mourning process is coming to terms with the loss of the person who has died, understanding and accepting that they are gone and will not return. Denial is common during this phase and some people may become stuck in the initial mourning phase.
2 **To process the pain of grief** – The pain experienced when grieving can be physical as well as emotional. Some people may try to avoid feeling pain and protect themselves from the effects of the loss. Feelings such as anxiety, depression, anger and loneliness are commonly experienced in grief.
3 **To adjust to a world without the deceased** – There are three elements of adjustment that need to be considered following the death of a loved one: internal (one's sense of self), external (how the death impacts on everyday functioning) and spiritual (impact on belief, values and perceptions of the world).
4 **To find an enduring connection with the deceased** while embarking on the journey of a life without them.

Worden (2018) believes the fourth stage is often the hardest to address and can take time to work through.

The tasks can be revisited over and over, and tasks can be worked through simultaneously, acknowledging that grief is a non-linear, fluid and complex process.

The dual-process model of coping with bereavement

Stroebe and Schut (2010) devised a two-stage model of bereavement which focuses on how people cope with loss. They believe that the bereaved alternate between two different kinds of coping: loss-oriented coping and restoration-oriented coping.

- Loss-oriented coping consists of processing the loss itself, during which the person may experience intrusive thoughts about the death.
- In the restoration-oriented phase, the bereaved will distract themselves from the grief by doing new things or developing a new hobby or skill.

Stroebe and Schut hypothesize that bereaved individuals fluctuate between the two phases, which is important to achieve adaptive coping.

Dealing with death by suicide

The World Health Organization (WHO) define suicide as 'the act of deliberately killing oneself' (WHO 2019). WHO report that around 800,000 people take their own life each year, and it was the second leading cause of death among 15–29 year olds globally in 2016. While suicide is a serious public health issue, prevention strategies involving timely, evidence-based interventions can be effective.

Suicide risk factors

There are many complex factors that are associated with an individual's increased risk of suicide. Underlying mental health disorders, gender, culture, youth or old age, financial status, substance misuse, previous attempts or a history of self-harm, abuse, adverse life events, access to lethal means, and a lack of healthcare support services are among the universal risk factors that have been identified. It is thought that a combination of these factors can further increase the risk of suicide and suicidal ideation (Chehil and Kutcher 2012).

While there are strong links between suicide and mental health disorders, WHO (2019) state that many suicides occur impulsively due to a loss of coping mechanisms in dealing with times of extreme stress, such as relationship break-downs, bereavement, financial hardship and long-term pain or serious illness diagnosis.

Rates of suicide are particularly high in vulnerable groups who encounter discrimination, such as refugees and migrants; indigenous groups; lesbian, gay, bisexual, transgender communities; and prisoners.

In most countries, death by suicide occurs more frequently in men than women. Reluctance to seek help, impulsive behaviour traits, and use of more lethal means are some of the factors associated with higher suicide rates in men compared to women. It is thought the biggest risk factor for both genders remains previous attempts at suicide (Chehil and Kutcher 2012).

Suicide prevention

Studies have shown that people do not actually want to die but they want the pain they are experiencing to end (Henden 2017). The National Suicide

Prevention Alliance (NSPA) is a network of public, private and voluntary organizations who focus on suicide prevention, taking a collective approach to reducing suicide and self-harm in England (NSPA 2021).

In 2012, the Coalition Government published a cross-government strategy for reducing suicide, which included six key objectives:

1 Reduce the risk of suicide in key high-risk groups
2 Tailor approaches to improve mental health in specific groups
3 Reduce access to the means of suicide
4 Provide better information and support to those bereaved or affected by suicide
5 Support the media in delivering sensitive approaches to suicide and suicidal behaviour
6 Support research, data collection and monitoring

The new strategy was implemented to reduce suicide rates and improve support for those affected by suicide. The strategy defines what government departments will do to contribute and bring together knowledge about higher risk groups, effective interventions and resources to support local action (HM Government and DOH 2012).

Suicide is a complex issue, and suicide prevention strategies require a collaborative approach across multiple sectors including health, education, agriculture, business, law, politics and the media. An integrated, coordinated response is required with a joint approach to make an impact on reducing suicide rates in the UK (WHO 2021). However, Platt and Niederkrotenthaler (2020) argue that the overall effectiveness of multisectoral approaches to suicide prevention remains questionable regarding efficacy and practicality of large-scale interventions, and further evidence-based research is ongoing.

Stigma and taboo

One of the challenges in suicide prevention remains the stigma that is associated with mental health problems, which can deter people from seeking and accessing the support that they need, which in turn increases isolation and suicide risk (Pitman et al. 2017).

Stigma around suicide stems back to the Middle Ages, where for centuries suicide was deemed a crime and viewed by the church as a sinful act. The phrase 'committed suicide' referred to the illegal act of taking one's own life, a term which in recent years has been abolished. In those days the remains of a person who died by suicide were destroyed to 'prevent the unleashing of evil spirits' and the family was ostracized, with no access to community support (Evans and Abrahamson 2020). Although this practice no longer occurs, there is still stigma surrounding suicide which is thought to impact on the grieving process and result in which will be discussed in this chapter. Pitman et al. (2017) conducted a study on data from people who experienced sudden bereavement through suicide and found that they felt highly stigmatized by the death, which can result in reluctance to seek support, putting them at greater risk of depression and suicide themselves. Families may experience a range of stigma-related perceptions such as shame, extreme guilt resulting from the belief that they could or should have prevented the death, a sense of rejection, lack of social support and a decrease in communication from friends and extended family (Sheehan et al. 2018). A reluctance by friends and family to talk about suicide, or not even acknowledging the death, may prevent the bereaved from sharing their feelings or seeking the support they need (Chapple et al. 2015).

A common misconception is that people with mental health conditions may be a danger to others, which is often compounded by the portrayal in the media or television. However, the most common mental health conditions do not have any links with violent or dangerous behaviour. The proportion of people living with a mental health problem who commit a violent crime is extremely low, and it is often because of alcohol or substance misuse. But the fear of being perceived as dangerous often means people are worried about talking about how they are feeling or accessing the help they need. The perception of taboo and stigma for the suicide bereaved has clear links with their reported experiences of complicated grief, depression and suicidal thoughts. Identifying suicide-related stigma, suicide postvention, evidence-based practice research, and anti-stigma campaigns should remain a priority in public health strategies (Chapple et al. 2015; Evans and Abrahamson 2020).

Suicide in the ambulance sector

In 2015, the National Ambulance Services' Medical Directors (NASMeD) highlighted the growing numbers of suicide deaths within UK ambulance services. Data from the Office for National Statistics (ONS) analysed between 2011 and 2015 showed that 75 per cent of male paramedics are at higher risk of suicide than any other group of healthcare professionals. The Association of Ambulance Chief Executives (AACE) commissioned a research study to investigate these concerns and provide recommendations for implementing a suicide prevention strategy.

AACE and the Office of the Chief Allied Health Professions Officer (CAHPO) launched three online publications in 2019 to provide support for mental health and well-being among the ambulance sector workforce with the aim of preventing the increasing prevalence of suicide. Multiple risk factors have been identified which impact on the health and well-being of ambulance staff, and a consensus statement sets out appropriate actions and recommendations for the prevention of suicide in ambulance services across the UK.

Complicated grief

Dealing with the death of a loved one is a devastating event which is followed by a period of bereavement. Some bereaved people develop prolonged and severe reactions to the loss, which can result in complicated grief (CG), estimated to affect 2–3 per cent of adults globally (Shoenberger et al. 2013). Complicated grief is more prevalent following sudden and unexpected deaths through trauma and suicide, and can present challenges which may not be seen in a non-traumatic or non-suicidal death. Complicated grief can increase the risk of developing mental health issues such as substance abuse, post-traumatic stress disorder (PTSD) and suicidal ideation, and an increased risk of cardio-vascular disease, cancer and hypertension. Complicated grief is defined by intense grief that lasts longer than the expected 'norm' and impacts on activities of daily living. Complicated grief can arise following any loss but has a prevalence of approximately 10–20 per cent after the death of a spouse and increases among parents suffering the loss of a child; it is less common following the death of a parent, grandparent, sibling or close friend (Shear 2015).

Cultural differences in dealing with death

Many people experience grief and a sense of loss after the death of a loved one. But the ways in which they experience and express these feelings may differ across cultures. Culture is a combination of beliefs, values, behaviours, traditions and rituals that members of a cultural group share. Each culture has its own rituals that influence the way in which grief is expressed. Observing cultural practices can provide a sense of belonging and comfort, and can also help those that are dying and bring reassurance to the loved ones who are preparing for their death. It is important to understand the various cultural and religious differences in dealing with death and bereavement, so that interventions are appropriate to the cultural context of the patients in our care (Parkes et al. 2015).

Each culture has a set of beliefs to understand the meaning of life and how death is approached. Some believe in an afterlife and look to the spirit of their loved one to influence their life, finding comfort in the notion that they are watching over them.

Rituals associated with death can have a positive impact on the grieving process and are a way for communities to support the bereaved. Rituals can provide structure and direct the mourners in the initial phases following a death. Rituals include how the deceased is cared for, who is present and what type of ceremony will be performed, such as burial or cremation. Some cultures cleanse and dress the body, express grief quietly in private or loudly in public such as 'wailing' or crying.

Another tradition shared by many cultures is wearing clothing that shows that they're grieving. Mourning dress such as black clothing, worn for a set period, may help communities prepare for the emotions displayed by the bereaved.

Beliefs and values can be adapted to meet individual needs and circumstances, and grief responses can vary within cultures. An example is societies made up of people from many backgrounds, developing their own unique customs and beliefs. The customs observed by one culture may be perceived as strange by another.

While it would be impossible to know all the cultural values, beliefs and customs associated with death, it is important to understand that there is no set way to mourn the loss of a loved one, and sensitivity and understanding is of paramount importance when caring for patients who are experiencing loss and grief.

Conclusion

Dealing with the death of a patient is an emotive and challenging aspect of paramedic practice and can be especially challenging in poignant deaths. Breaking bad news to loved ones in the unpredictable pre-hospital environment poses further challenges, and using a model or clear structure to deliver the news, while considering the impact that the news will have, can help to ensure an effective approach.

Understanding reactions, responses and the normal process of grief can equip the paramedic with the skills required to effectively manage those suffering the devastating loss of a loved one. Recognizing risk factors for the potential of developing complicated grief is important when considering referral pathways for the bereaved, particularly following suicide and traumatic deaths.

Effective communication is one of the most important attributes a paramedic must possess, particularly when breaking bad news; how the news is communicated is as important as the news itself.

As well as providing emotional support to patients and their loved ones, it is of vital importance that paramedics maintain their own mental health and well-being to be able to provide that support.

References

Bowlby, J. (1973) *Attachment and Loss*. London: Hogarth Press.

Bowyer, M.W., Hanson, J.L., Pimentel, E.A. et al. (2010) Teaching breaking bad news using mixed reality simulation, *Journal of Surgical Research*, 159(1): 462–7. doi:10.1016/j.jss.2009.04.032.

Buglass, E. (2010) Grief and bereavement theories, *Nursing Standard*, 24(41): 44–7.

Chapple, A., Ziebland, S. and Hawton, K. (2015) Taboo and the different death? Perceptions of those bereaved by suicide or other traumatic death, *Sociology of Health & Illness*, 37(4): 610–25.

Chehil, S. and Kutcher, S.P. (2012) *Suicide Risk Management: A Manual for Health Professionals*. Hoboken, NJ: John Wiley & Sons.

Cole, A. (2019) Breaking bad news, *Optometry Today*, 59(1): 67.

Evans, A. and Abrahamson, K. (2020) The influence of stigma on suicide bereavement: A systematic review, *Journal of Psychosocial Nursing and Mental Health Services*, 58(4): 21–7.

Henden, J. (2017) *Preventing Suicide: The Solution Focused Approach*. Hoboken, NJ: John Wiley & Sons.

HM Government and Department of Health (2012) *Preventing Suicide in England: A Cross-government Outcomes Strategy to Save Lives*. London: HM Government. Available at: https://assets.publishing.service.gov.uk/government/uploads/system/uploads/attachment_data/file/430720/Preventing-Suicide-.pdf (accessed 24 August 2021).

Hobgood, C., Mathew, D., Woodyard, D.J., Shofer, F.S. and Brice, J.H. (2013) Death in the field: Teaching paramedics to deliver effective death notifications using the educational intervention 'GRIEV_ING', *Prehospital Emergency Care*, 17(4): 501–10.

Iserson, K. (2000) Notifying survivors about sudden, unexpected deaths, *Western Journal of Medicine*, 173(4): 261–5.

Isokääntä, S., Koivula, K., Honkalampi, K., Kokki, H. and Cravero, J. (2019) Resilience in children and their parents enduring pediatric medical traumatic stress, *Pediatric Anesthesia*, 29(3): 218–25.

Keefe-Cooperman, K. and Brady-Amoon, P. (2013) Breaking bad news in counselling: Applying the PEWTER model in the school setting, *Journal of Creativity in Mental Health*, 8(3): 265–77. doi: 10.1080/15401383.2013.821926.

Kubler-Ross, E. (1969) *On Death and Dying*. New York: Springer.

Liddicoat, P. (2018) Breaking bad news, *InnovAiT*, 11(12): 671–5.

Marschollek, P., Bąkowska, K., Bąkowski, W., Marschollek, K. and Tarkowski, R. (2019) Oncologists and breaking bad news – from the informed patients' point of view. The Evaluation of the SPIKES protocol implementation, *Journal of Cancer Education*, 34(2): 375-380.

Maunder, E. and Maguire, D. (2017) Breaking bad news: The need for a coping mechanism in paramedicine, *International Paramedic Practice*, 7(1): 3–7.

MIND (2016) *Blue Light Programme Research Summary: An Evaluation of the Impact of our Mental Health Support for Emergency Services Staff and Volunteers in 2015 to 2016*. London: MIND.

Mitchell, A.M., Wesner, S., Brownson, L., Gale, D.D., Garand, L. and Havill, A. (2006) Effective communication with bereaved child survivors of suicide, *Journal of Child and Adolescent Psychiatric Nursing*, 19(3): 130–6.

Mowll, J. (2007) Reality and regret, *Bereavement Care*, 26(1): 3–6. doi: 10.1080/02682620708657676.

Narayanan, V., Bista, B. and Koshy, C. (2010). 'BREAKS' protocol for breaking bad news, *Indian Journal of Palliative Care*, 16(2): 61–5.

National Suicide Prevention Alliance (NSPA) (2021) *Strategic Framework 2019–2021*. Surrey: NSPA. Available at: https://nspa.org.uk/wp-content/uploads/2021/07/NSPA-Strategic-framework-2019-2021_WEB.pdf (accessed 24 August 2021).

Park, I., Gupta, A., Mandani, K., Haubner, L. and Peckler, B. (2010) Breaking bad news education for emergency medicine residents: A novel training module using simulation with the SPIKES protocol, *Journal of Emergencies, Trauma and Shock*, 3(4): 385–8.

Parkes, C.M., Laungani, P. and Young, B. (2015) *Death and Bereavement Across Cultures*, 2nd edn. London: Routledge.

Pitman, A., Rantell, K., Marston, L., King, M. and Osborn, D. (2017) Perceived stigma of sudden bereavement as a risk factor for suicidal thoughts and suicide attempt: Analysis of British cross-sectional survey data on 3387 young bereaved adults, *International Journal of Environmental Research and Public Health*, 14(3): 286.

Platt, S. and Niederkrotenthaler, T. (2020) Suicide prevention programs: Evidence base and best practice, *Crisis : The Journal of Crisis Intervention and Suicide Prevention*, 41(S1): S99–S124.

Reny, D., Root, S., Chreiman, K., Browning, R. and Sims, C. (2020) A body of evidence: Barriers to family viewing after death by gun violence, *Journal of Surgical Research*, 247: 556–62.

Shear, M.K. (2015) Complicated grief, *New England Journal of Medicine*, 372(2): 153–60.

Sheehan, L., Corrigan, P.W., Al-Khouja, M.A. et al. (2018) Behind closed doors: The stigma of suicide loss survivors, *Omega: Journal of Death and Dying*, 77(4): 330–49.

Shoenberger, J.M., Yeghiazarian, S., Rios, C. and Henderson, S.O. (2013) Death notification in the emergency department: Survivors and physicians, *Western Journal of Emergency Medicine*, 14(2): 181–5.

Stroebe, M.S. and Schut, H.A.W. (2010) The dual process model of coping with bereavement: A decade on, *Omega: Journal of Death and Dying*, 61(4): 273–89.

Tan, K.K., Pang, A. and Kang, J.X. (2019) Breaking bad news with CONSOLE: Toward a framework integrating medical protocols with crisis communication, *Public Relations Review*, 45(1): 153–66.

Tuffrey-Wijne, I. and Rose, T. (2017) Investigating the factors that affect the communication of death-related bad news to people with intellectual disabilities by staff in residential and supported living services: An interview study, *Journal of Intellectual Disability Research*, 61(8): 727–36.

Villagran, M., Goldsmith, J., Wittenberg-Lyles, E. and Baldwin, P. (2010) Creating COMFORT: A communication-based model for breaking bad news, *Communication Education*, 59(3): 220–34.

Walker, E. (2018) Death notification delivery and training methods, *Journal of Paramedic Practice*, 10(8): 334–41.

Worden, J.W. (2018) *Grief Counseling and Grief Therapy: A Handbook for the Mental Health Practitioner*, 5th edn. New York: Springer.

World Health Organization (WHO) (2021) *Suicide* factsheet, WHO website. Available at: https://www.who.int/news-room/fact-sheets/detail/suicide (accessed 24 August 2021).

9 | Trauma-informed care

Jo Augustus

Learning objectives

- Recognize the causes and characteristics of post-traumatic stress disorder
- Consider evidence-based interventions for post-traumatic stress disorder
- Discuss decision-making processes in pre-hospital care
- Analyse research specific to post-traumatic stress disorder in paramedics
- Consider the international contexts of emergency medicine and post-traumatic stress disorder
- Understand what trauma-informed care is in organizational contexts

Introduction

Trauma-informed care is an evidence-based universal approach to the delivery of care that aims to understand the implications of trauma for both the individual and providers of healthcare (Isobel and Edwards 2017; Oral et al. 2020). Here trauma is referred to as both the psychological and physical impacts relating to distressing events such as road traffic accidents or exposure to violence. From a diagnostic perspective this relates to post-traumatic stress disorder (PTSD), which is explored in section 9.3. In the absence of taking a trauma-informed care approach there is a recognition that healthcare providers will adopt task-oriented and problem-focused care, which is far removed from person-centred care practices (Isobel and Edwards 2017). Person-centred care practices are essential in all aspects of the recovery journey of an individual, from the first point of contact with healthcare professionals. As a framework, trauma-informed care may also offer recommendations for managing workforce stress and distress. Therefore, the authors are proposing that a trauma-informed care approach is an essential part of pre-hospital care and so is integral to the role of a paramedic. The following will explore what trauma-informed care is and its relevance for pre-hospital care.

Trauma-informed care practices

The historical context of trauma-informed care

Trauma-informed care emerged as a strengths-based approach in the post-war period in response to the changing needs of the clinical population. The trauma-informed model of care highlights the need for individual practitioners and organizations to recognize both the prevalence and impact of trauma. Through this recognition, service provision will become more trauma aware.

Historically, the way society has viewed trauma has often been captured in reference to industrial change or warfare (Lasiuk and Hegadoren 2006). The onset of the Industrial Revolution in the eighteenth century led to an increase in catastrophic accidents. These are documented in the form of industrial accidents, such as those in factories. In addition, the changing nature of warfare saw the development of different trauma-related problems and how trauma was viewed by society. For example, the use of heavy explosives in the First World War related symptoms to 'shell shock', and during the Second World War the term 'morale weakness' was attributed to soldiers who were seen as having personality flaws (Benedek and Ursano 2009; Center for Substance Abuse Treatment 2014). In addition, during the Second World War the phrase 'battle fatigue' began the recognition that soldiers required time to rest in between battles. However, it wasn't until the Korean and Vietnam Wars that there became a focus on talking therapies as a clinical intervention. Here the concept of group therapies was born and used as a treatment for post-traumatic stress disorder. Alongside this the third edition of the Diagnostic and Statistical Manual of Mental Disorders published in 1980 (DSM-III) introduced post-traumatic stress disorder as a diagnosis and classified it as an anxiety disorder (Lasiuk and Hegadoren 2006). The diagnosis required the experience of a specific stressor, e.g. something catastrophic, that is characterized as outside of what is deemed a normal human experience (APA 1980). This triggered a growing body of research specific to trauma and a shift in approaches to recovery, which Information Box 9.1 explores (Center for Substance Abuse Treatment 2014).

Information box 9.1 Historical shifts in trauma treatment

First wave trauma treatment

The first wave of trauma treatment was characterized by a focus on symptom management to promote recovery and increase daily functioning. Not only was there a recognition of PTSD as a collection of symptoms, there was also a sense of the impact it has on everyday life activities. This saw the development of group-based interventions that then diversified to include individuals outside of warfare, such as people affected by natural disasters. This required further developments in approaches to trauma treatment: second wave trauma.

Second wave trauma treatment

The second wave in trauma treatment was characterized by psychosocial approaches, that included psycho-education and empowerment. These were designed as an alternative to clinical interventions, not to replace them but rather to operate alongside. Here the focus was on both peer support, delivered as a group, and self-sustaining models of recovery. Such psychosocial educational and empowerment approaches were designed to manage trauma symptoms and in doing so provide a social context for trauma management. Here there was a recognition that in order to be effective a trauma-informed approach was required, at an organizational or programme level.

Third wave trauma treatment

The third wave in trauma treatment saw a fundamental shift away from a deficit-based to a strengths-based model of care, termed trauma-informed care. In addition, this model sought to empower individuals to seek their own recovery journey, supported by a particular service provider. This approach may adopt a model of recovery that is made up of goals or actions defined by the individual. Here a working with, or in partnership with, approach is adopted as a way to support recovery. Such a psychosocial empowerment partnership provides person-centred care and is deemed effective at moving away from traditional top-down medicalized approaches to recovery.

Adapted from Salasin (2011) and Center for Substance Abuse Treatment (2014).

By shifting away from a deficit-based approach towards a strengths-based model, an individualized approach can be taken that reduces labelling and arguably associated stigma. Rather than labelling an individual's behaviour as challenging, the function of behaviour can be explored and addressed. This approach seeks to adopt a social perspective, where every behaviour is a form of communication: in other words a reaction to a trigger such as distress (Wilson and Beresford 2002). Through addressing the distress, the individual can be free of old patterns of behaviour that may be deemed harmful. In addition, if behaviour is not labelled as challenging, then it may be met with less intrusive interventions (Sweeney et al. 2016). Case Study 9.1 explores this concept through the lens of a paramedic.

Case study 9.1

Marianne is well known to the local emergency services through repeated call-outs made by her, her family and on occasion her neighbours. Typically, early evening she overdoses on over the counter and prescription medication, which she consumes with large amounts of alcohol. This is with the intent of ending her life. The frequency of this varies, although it worsens near Christmas. As she sobers up she realizes the consequences of her action and dials 999 requesting paramedics. On other occasions her mum and sister, on returning home, have found her unconscious and subsequently called an ambulance. Less frequently, the neighbours have called the police on witnessing Marianne with what appears to be a weapon, shouting outside her home. Marianne can occasionally be verbally aggressive and uncooperative towards others trying to help her, especially paramedics on site. The paramedics who know Marianne well often label her as difficult, manipulative and a time waster. They often tease each other about who will get the call-out this week. Marianne is 39 years old, overweight and a heavy smoker.

Pause for thought: What are some of the identified risk factors that need to be considered here? What might be the mental health diagnosis based on what we know about Marianne? What do you predict might be possible outcomes for Marianne?

A trauma-informed approach to Case study 9.1: Marianne

Karl is a paramedic who transferred to the local ambulance service having recently moved house to be nearer his family. He is on shift with Kerry who knows Marianne well and gives Karl a potted history of her recent contacts. Karl approaches Marianne, who is subdued, and introduces himself as the newbie. Karl continues with his assessment, and while taking observations asks Marianne when this started happening and what might have triggered it in the first place. Marianne discloses that she was attacked and gang raped by a group of men dressed in a type of uniform in the early evening, around five years ago on the way home from a works Christmas party. She was also sexually abused as a child. Karl goes on to ask if Marianne knows what led to her overdosing and drinking alcohol. Marianne explained that as it gets dark she often relives the gang rape and believes they will do it again, as they were not prosecuted due to a lack of evidence. To cope with this, Marianne uses substances to reduce the reliving although she knows it just makes her angry. Karl explained what he was going to do next, including taking her to A&E for treatment, and asked if that was ok with her. He encouraged her to speak to the mental health liaison nurse in A&E about being referred for talking therapy, to reduce the impact of the reliving she experiences. Marianne didn't know what this meant and asked Karl to speak to the A&E staff.

Case study conclusions

A trauma-informed approach shifts conversations from 'what's wrong' to 'what happened'. Fundamentally this can shift the emphasis to what is happening for the individual in the present, in order to engage in available resources. In the example of Marianne this meant using gentle questioning, active listening and clear communication to consider alternative pathways.

Pause for thought: What questions did Karl pose? What variables might be present when assessing Marianne? How might these variables be mitigated?

NB: The authors recognize there are a number of variables here, however adopting a strengths-based approach can lead to positive change on an individual's recovery journey.

Trauma-informed care seeks to reframe thinking about a situation differently, focusing attention on the complexity of behaviour by understanding its function (Harris and Fallot 2001). As a consequence, other possibilities may be presented, enabling the individual to develop alternative coping strategies using additional resources available to them. Here the individual shifts towards becoming a survivor. This arguably adopts a relapse prevention approach (Sweeney et al. 2016).

Considerations in communication

There can often be fear associated with talking about trauma, a sense of retraumatizing the individual, perhaps through a lack of appropriate training (Read et al. 2007). However, trauma-informed care approaches retraumatization respectfully, recognizing the benefits of telling the individual's trauma narrative in a way that offers possibilities of change (Filson 2011). The individual survivor has a choice not to construct their narrative at that time, and if they do choose to do so it is conducted at their pace, while being listened to, as well as being offered support afterwards. Here a whole person approach is taken by all aspects of the organization, which is achieved by offering ongoing staff training and support (Sweeney et al. 2016). In doing this there exists a shared responsibility between staff and individual survivors. The relationships within the organizational environment become of central importance and act as agents of change. Individuals may be referred to specialist services for additional support (Sweeney et al. 2016). As discussed in the case study, it is hoped that Marianne will access such support in the near future to prevent the need for further pre-hospital care and hospital admissions.

Trauma-informed care seeks to reduce, or indeed remove altogether, the use of control and coercion such as medication as a restraint. Here the least restrictive option is applied and staff are supported to consistently offer this as a first-line intervention. Here there is an understanding that power can lead to revictimization, whereas collaboration and trust can become central tenets of change. For this to be effectively applied, training and support must be across the multidisciplinary team, including paramedics (Sweeney et al. 2016).

Information box 9.2 Adverse childhood experiences

Research has documented that adverse childhood experiences (ACEs) increase the risk of poor health outcomes in later life (Shonkoff et al. 2012; Sun et al. 2017). ACEs include being exposed to physical, emotional or sexual abuse, emotional or physical neglect, witnessing a maternal figure being abused or having an incarcerated parent, parental divorce, living with an individual who is depressed and living with an individual who used substances (Mersky et al. 2013). These traumatic experiences are linked to lifelong negative mental and physical health outcomes, including chronic disease, depression and risk for attempted suicide. These outcomes can occur in different ways, including leading to inflammation, activating an allostatic response to stress that impacts on the immune, nervous and endocrine systems (Danese et al. 2009; Danese and McEwen 2012). Epigenetics also plays a role in the context of heritable changes in genome function, where trauma can act to modify gene expression in the prefrontal cortex (Anacker et al. 2014). These negative outcomes can have a profound impact on the individual's functioning, including roles and responsibilities, such as parenting (Mersky et al. 2013; Lomanowska et al. 2017; Sun et al. 2017). Such findings require targeted programmes to prevent and minimize the impact of ACEs.

The principles of trauma-informed care

Trauma-informed care offers a whole person, strengths-based approach and supportive framework, to engage individuals who have a history of trauma. Central to this is the need to learn the core principles and practices of trauma-informed care, through ongoing provision of training and supervisory structures.

There are four principles (Herman and Whitaker 2020):

1 A recognition of the high prevalence and impact of trauma, as well as the capacity to change and recover, for individuals, families and the wider community
2 An understanding of the symptoms associated with trauma in those accessing services
3 The provision of a responsive service that integrates knowledge about trauma into all levels of organizational practices, including policy and procedure
4 Reducing the likelihood of unintentional retraumatization, that can occur as a result of non-trauma-informed organizational practices

There is a recognition that a trauma-informed care approach could act to improve the levels of workforce satisfaction. For these principles to be implemented effectively, there is a need to continually evaluate and develop services provision, in order to sustain a trauma-informed workforce (Center for Substance Abuse Treatment 2014; Herman and Whitaker 2020).

Information box 9.3 Pre-hospital care: children and young people

Research has shown that treating children can be stressful for the attending paramedics (Gunnarsson and Stomberg 2009; Avraham et al. 2014; Nordén et al. 2014; Öberg et al. 2015; Alisic et al. 2017). This may relate to a lack of training or experience due to infrequent call-outs that involve children, coupled with the high risk they may be presented with (Cottrell et al. 2014). In addition, children may find such treatment traumatic, as well as their family members, which in turn may result in a diagnosis of PTSD or acute stress disorder. Therefore, the role of the paramedic is crucial in minimizing the impact of the traumatic experience. Research studies have indicated that a child's outcomes seem to relate to the initial experiences, including those of both threat, distress and the support received (Alisic et al. 2011; Trickey et al. 2012; Marsac et al. 2014).

Case study 9.2

Callum sustained dental trauma following a scooter accident, fracturing both front upper incisors. Callum is 9 years old. He was taken by ambulance to the emergency dental unit at the local paediatric hospital. Understandably distressed and in a lot of pain, he was met with friendly reassuring staff who assessed the extent of the injury and administered paracetamol for his pain. The assessment established that both teeth were significantly damaged, requiring extensive dental treatment over a number of months. Callum was subsequently discharged from hospital and it was arranged for him to return the following week to commence treatment.

During the first appointment, Callum was informed of the process and staff took time to explain in simple terms what would happen, ensuring every step of the procedure was fully described to Callum and his parents. Callum was anxious and became distressed when the anaesthetic was administered. It appeared that some of the distress related to a previous negative experience at the dentist. He explained his anxieties and was reassured that the anaesthetic would take all of his pain away.

While the dentist was drilling into the root canal, Callum indicated he wished to stop, becoming distressed and verbalizing extreme pain. He was told there was no pain and the procedure would be over soon. He continued to cry throughout the remainder of the treatment, and when it was over he leapt out of the chair and into the corridor outside. For the next few treatments Callum began to be aggressive, refusing to travel to the hospital and becoming obstructive and uncooperative with the staff. During some appointments he refused to sit in the dentist's chair and the appointment had to be cancelled. However, it remained essential that Callum underwent all of the treatment in order to save his teeth. The treatment was finally completed after two long years.

Pause for thought: Having read Callum's case study, what could have been done differently by staff? In addition, what were some of the positive experiences of Callum's interactions with hospital staff? Finally, consider how these skills could be transferable to pre-hospital care.

Why did Callum react so badly?

He hadn't felt listened to. He was promised there would be no pain and there was. He wasn't given any further anaesthesia as it was deemed unnecessary. He stopped trusting the staff and the relationship between patient and clinician broke down. He was too young to articulate his feelings, and his anxiety and fear manifested in his subsequent behaviour.

What could be done differently?

It is important to listen to a patient's anxieties and concerns, and not to promise there will be no pain where there is a chance there might be. Callum had a high tolerance to anaesthesia, which was not considered due to his age. His previous experiences had not been acknowledged, resulting in a procedure he had been assured would be pain-free causing pain and distress and an enduring fear of the dentist.

Alisic et al. (2017) proposes two different guidelines to reduce trauma symptoms, as well as improving self-efficacy: firstly the psychological model of first aid, and secondly the distress, emotional and family (DEF) protocol, which the Information Box 9.4 summarizes (Brymer et al. 2006; Stuber et al. 2006).

Information box 9.4 Psychological first aid model

1 Initial interaction and engagement
2 Providing safety and comfort
3 Stabilization
4 Collating information regarding current needs and concerns
5 Provision of practical support
6 Encouraging connection with social support networks
7 Information specific to coping strategies
8 Connecting with and or signposting to collaborative services

Distress, emotion and family protocol

Following the assessment and treatment of physical health needs, the protocol suggests the following be addressed:

D – the distress of the patient
E – the provision of emotional support for the patient
F – consideration of the family

Adapted from Alisic et al. (2017)

The psychological first aid model provides eight steps that can be adapted depending on the needs of the individual (Brymer et al. 2006). The distress, emotion and family protocol has three components and can precede the airway, breathing and circulation model (Stuber et al. 2006; Kassam-Adams et al. 2013). The DEF protocol also provides guidance specific to children (Alisic et al. 2017). Arguably both approaches are focused on the period after a traumatic event, however consideration can be given to each during treatment. Both approaches may help in the implementation of trauma-informed care during pre-hospital care (Magruder et al. 2016).

Causes of trauma in pre-hospital care

There is an acknowledgement that individuals receiving mental health treatment are more likely to experience trauma. Broadly, this forms the basis of trauma-informed care (Isobel and Edwards 2017). Trauma can result from a number of different factors specific to pre-hospital care; this can include interpersonal interactions that can lead to the individual feeling disempowered or neglected, and may relate to previous patterns experienced in that person's lifetime. Another consideration is that of clinical staff who are regularly exposed to trauma and may also have experienced feelings of being disempowered. This can lead to the clinician feeling unable to manage the trauma presented to them, with an unintended consequence of retraumatization. Arguably, given the significant impact this can have on individuals, their families and communities, it is the organization's responsibility to create environments that are trauma-informed. Trauma-informed care could offer a model of psychological safety while reducing harm caused through any examination or treatment. Therefore, there is an opportunity to apply a model of trauma-informed care alongside existing pre-hospital care approaches used by paramedics.

Diagnosis: post-traumatic stress disorder

As a mental health diagnosis, post-traumatic stress disorder (PTSD) is closely associated with poor health outcomes, including mental health comorbidity and usage of healthcare services, reduced physical health and subsequently quality of life, as well as early death (Greene et al. 2016; Lehavot et al. 2018). Therefore it remains important on the political agenda as well as a consideration for all organizations.

Risk factors

When looking at any diagnosis, it is important to consider the risk factors involved. In other words, while anyone could develop PTSD, there are factors that may increase the likelihood of developing the condition. Typically, this looks at the interactions between genetic, biological, psychological and social risk factors. More specific risk factors include adverse childhood experiences, poor social support, a previous psychiatric disorder, psychological inflexibility and low educational achievement (Williamson and Greenberg 2019).

Diagnosis: signs and symptoms

PTSD may develop after being exposed to a perceived or actual life-threatening event or series of events. In order to meet the diagnostic criteria, symptoms must be persistent for at least several weeks and induce significant impairment in all areas of functioning. It is characterized by the following (World Health Organization 2018; Williamson and Greenberg 2019):

1 Re-experiencing the event or events as if they are occurring in the present, typified by intrusive memories, flashbacks or nightmares. This may occur as one or more sensory experiences and is usually coupled with overwhelming emotions, in particular fear or terror and physical sensations.
2 Avoidance of thinking about or remembering the event or activities, situation or individuals associated with the event or events.
3 A persistent sense of heightened current threat, such as being hypervigilant or easily startled.

Of note is that the event or series of events is experienced as extremely threatening or horrific. In addition, the event(s) could be experienced through direct contact, being a witness to or learning about it indirectly from someone else. In a professional context one could also be repeatedly exposed to traumatic events directly or indirectly (Williamson and Greenberg 2019).

There are exclusions from this diagnosis, including acute stress disorder and complex post-traumatic stress disorder, which Information Box 9.5 briefly explores.

Information box 9.5 Acute stress disorder

Acute stress disorder is the development of short-lived cognitive, emotional, somatic or behavioural symptoms that result from extremely threatening or horrific events. Such events include natural disasters, war and assault. This may include symptoms specific to anxiety, e.g. tachycardia. This is considered a normal response to the particular event and typically subsides within a few days following the event or after threatening or horrific events have ceased (World Health Organization 2018).

Complex post-traumatic stress disorder

Complex post-traumatic stress disorder (CPTSD) may develop further to exposure to extremely threatening or horrific events that are typically persistent or prolonged and escape is difficult. Examples may include domestic violence, childhood abuse or torture. In addition to meeting the PTSD diagnostic criteria CPTSD includes:

1 Difficulty regulating emotion
2 Reduced self-belief, with feelings of guilt, shame or failure
3 Interpersonal difficulties such as problems having meaningful relationships

These symptoms induce impairment in all areas of functioning (World Health Organization 2018; Williamson and Greenberg 2019).

NB: Where these symptoms occur but there is little or no impairment of functioning and PTSD diagnostic criteria is not met, other diagnoses may be relevant. Here a recommended referral to a mental health professional such as a psychiatrist may be appropriate.

Case study 9.3 Post-traumatic stress disorder

John is well known to the local ambulance service since his discharge from the military five years ago. He had served for 12 years and was medically discharged after receiving a serious abdominal wound while on operation with his section. It was thought his friend triggered a roadside improvised explosive device (IED). Two of his close friends died. He required over seven different surgeries, of which two were done under emergency conditions. John began using alcohol to cope, drinking increasing amounts and on a regular basis. This often leads to fights at his local pub, resulting in his wounds needing medical attention. On other occasions he disappears for days at a time, sleeping near the local quarry, and on being found he often has unexplained physical injuries. He has expressed survivors' guilt and suicidal ideation although thoughts of his mum stop him ending his life.

Questions to ask:

Have you been experiencing flashbacks of your time in the military? How often do these happen?

Have you ever had any psychological support?

Pause for reflection: By asking these questions, what difference might this make to John? As a paramedic have you got any concerns about asking John about his trauma?

Information box 9.6 Health outcomes: cardiometabolic diseases

Research conducted over many years has explored the link between PTSD and poor health outcomes (Koenen et al. 2017). Findings suggest that PTSD can lead to a variety of physical health problems, including cardiometabolic diseases, of which cardiovascular disease and type 2 diabetes are considered particular risks (Vaccarino et al. 2014; Lohr et al. 2015; Roberts et al. 2015). However, despite this evidence PTSD is not noted as a risk factor within the medical fields of cardiovascular or endocrinology. More compelling evidence is required to demonstrate that PTSD causally contributes to cardiometabolic diseases (Koenen et al. 2017).

Pre-hospital delay: acute coronary syndrome

The link between a delay from symptom onset to hospital presentation for acute coronary syndrome and poor clinical outcomes is well researched (Ting et al. 2008, 2010; Smolderen et al. 2010). Research links PTSD as a risk factor to cardiovascular disease and it is also associated with poor outcomes after a myocardial infarction (Shemesh et al. 2004; Kubzansky et al. 2007; Walczewska et al. 2010; Ahmadi et al. 2011). De Luca et al. (2004) recognize the clinical implications of delays on mortality rates. Avoidance is a key characteristic of PTSD, so it is possible that patients may actively delay seeking assessment at the point of onset of cardiac symptoms. In addition, patients may also mistake cardiac symptoms for those of PTSD. Individuals presenting with acute coronary syndrome as well as PTSD symptoms were associated with longer pre-hospital delays (Newman et al. 2011). Although there are known non-modifiable covariates (e.g. age, gender, race), there are also many psychosocial variables that are modifiable, which could be addressed to reduce the delays. While more research is required into this area, there is evidence to indicate that these delays need addressing to minimize impact on health outcomes.

Interventions

Treatment

Following exposure to a traumatic event, an evidence-based intervention is not encouraged within the first month. This is largely because symptoms are expected to resolve on their own within a month. In addition, using trauma counselling or psychological debriefing within the first month is recognized as a contraindicator, increasing the possibility of the individual experiencing mental health difficulties longer term. Alternatively, the individual could be encouraged to access social support and temporarily reduce exposure to stressors associated with the trauma. Distress should also be monitored within the first month, following exposure to trauma. This will enable the individual to develop an awareness of the intensity of their distress symptoms and inform whether further psychological therapy is needed (Bisson 2007; Williamson and Greenberg 2019).

Information box 9.7 Prevalence of PTSD

Approximately one in three people in the UK report experiencing a significant traumatic event during the course of their life, although this figure is probably considerably higher for those working in trauma-exposed occupations or in many health-related professions, and in less developed countries where trauma is more commonplace.

Research indicates that PTSD is common, although it is important to note that not all individuals who experience trauma will go on to develop PTSD. The prevalence of PTSD in the UK is approximately 4.4 per cent, with frequently more than 80 per cent comorbidity (Fear et al. 2016; Williamson and Greenberg 2019). Prevalence is likely to be significantly greater for individuals working in occupations where trauma exposure is higher, such as the military and emergency services. For example, prevalence rates increase up to 20 per cent for ambulance workers (Fear et al. 2016; Williamson and Greenberg 2019). Therefore, it is an essential priority for ambulance services to support their employees through a model of trauma-informed care.

The National Institute for Health and Care Excellence (NICE) recommends different psychological interventions in the treatment of PTSD (NICE 2018). These include trauma-focused cognitive behavioural therapy (TF-CBT) and eye movement desensitization and reprocessing (EMDR). Figure 9.1 shows the NICE guidelines flow chart for treating adults with a diagnosis of PTSD.

The flow chart in Figure 9.1 depicts the care pathway for individuals with PTSD. Individuals would usually be offered either TF-CBT or EMDR, however this depends on the service provision and what training therapists have received (NICE 2018). Although EMDR is offered routinely, it is possible that TF-CBT is more frequently offered in practice. Both treatments are provided through weekly sessions, over eight to twelve weeks, however more should be provided if multiple traumas are present (NICE 2018). Note that TF-CBT tends to be delivered as an hour-long session, whereas EMDR is typically an hour and a half. Medication is not routinely offered as an initial intervention, but it may be used to treat comorbidities if the patient chooses this. The following sections will explore TF-CBT and EMDR in more detail (Williamson and Greenberg 2019).

Trauma-focused cognitive behaviour therapy

CBT is usually comprised of four components: psycho-education, anxiety management, exposure to the feared situation and cognitive restructuring. In line with NICE guidance, trauma-focused cognitive behaviour therapy (TF-CBT) interventions include:

Figure 9.1 NICE guidelines flow chart for treating adults with a diagnosis of PTSD

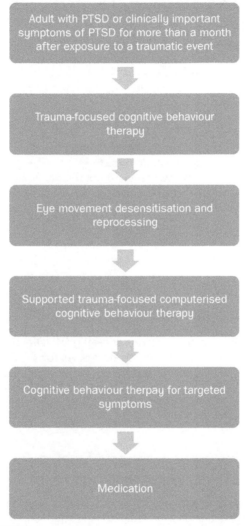

Adult with PTSD or clinically important symptoms of PTSD for more than a month after exposure to a traumatic event

Trauma-focused cognitive behaviour therapy

Eye movement desensitisation and reprocessing

Supported trauma-focused computerised cognitive behaviour therapy

Cognitive behaviour therpay for targeted symptoms

Medication

Adapted from NICE (2018)

- cognitive processing therapy
- cognitive therapy for PTSD
- narrative exposure therapy
- prolonged exposure therapy

In addition, NICE guidance stipulates that TF-CBT intervention should be based on an evidence-based protocol and should be provided by an appropriately trained practitioner who receives ongoing supervision. Information Box 9.8 summarizes components of the intervention that should be included.

Information box 9.8 Components of the TF-CBT intervention for adults

- Provide psycho-education about the individual's reactions to trauma, as well as offering strategies for managing arousal to triggers and flashbacks of the trauma, and safety planning.
- Include elaborating on the trauma memory and actually processing the trauma memories.
- Include processing trauma-related emotions, which may include shame, guilt, loss and anger.
- Involve restructuring the meaning of the trauma memory for the individual, which may include opportunity for growth.
- Provide help to overcome avoidance of the trauma or situation.
- Focus on re-establishing adaptive functioning, which may include work and social relationships.
- Prepare for treatment ending, which may include additional top-up sessions if needed.

(Adapted from NICE 2018)

Eye movement desensitization and reprocessing

Eye movement desensitization and reprocessing (EMDR) is an evidence-based protocol involving a number of specific stages. As for TF-CBT, NICE guidance stipulates that EMDR should be based on an evidence-based protocol and should be provided by an appropriately trained practitioner who receives ongoing supervision (NICE 2018). These stages are summarized in Information Box 9.9.

Information box 9.9 Stages of EMDR intervention for adults

- Provide psycho-education about the individual's reactions to trauma, as well as managing distressing memories and situations.
- Identify and treat targeted memories (e.g. these are often visual images) and promote alternative positive beliefs focused on self.
- Use in-session bilateral stimulation for the targeted memories until they are no longer distressing. This is usually with eye movements, however other methods of bilateral stimulation can be used to adapt to the needs of the client.
- The introduction of techniques for self-calming and/or managing flashbacks should also be included to support clients both in the session and between sessions.

(Adapted from Shapiro 2001; NICE 2018)

Pre-hospital care and decision-making

As discussed earlier, PTSD symptoms are a common occurrence in some physical health problems, including acute respiratory distress syndrome (ARDS). Research has found that survivors of ARDS and other critical illnesses commonly experience PTSD (Bienvenu et al. 2013, 2018; Parker et al. 2015; Jackson et al. 2016; Hosey et al. 2019). Interestingly, results showed that mild sedation, illness severity and length of stay in intensive care were not connected to PTSD. For these patients, PTSD risk factors were associated with a pre-existing mental health diagnosis, and the use of benzodiazepines while in intensive care (Davydow et al. 2008; Parker et al. 2015; Huang et al. 2016; Bienvenu et al. 2018; Devlin et al. 2018; Hosey et al. 2019). In reference to non-hospitalization, research conducted by Einvik et al. (2021) found additional risk factors led to patients developing PTSD. Individuals who were not hospitalized, and had a previous diagnosis of depression and severe COVID-19 symptoms, experienced PTSD symptoms. Here there is a recognition that dyspnoea and overall symptom load leads to an increased risk of experiencing PTSD symptoms. Therefore, from a pre-hospital care perspective there is a need to consider the treatment being used in order to reduce the risk of the patient developing PTSD. This may include considering the least intrusive intervention while maintaining the patient's safety.

Pause for reflection: What might the least intrusive, first-line intervention be in pre-hospital care?

What might your role be or not be in advising the patient?

Information box 9.10 Post-traumatic stress disorder and psychosis

Individuals with a diagnosis of psychosis are frequently found to experience trauma, following the increased risk of being exposed to traumatic events (Lommen and Restifo 2009; Swan et al. 2017). This can be caused by a variety of bio-psycho-social factors – for example, victimization rates are higher for individuals with a severe and enduring mental health problem such as psychosis, when compared to the general population (Maniglio 2009). Social factors are also an important consideration, such as isolation or limited access to resources that may lead to poverty. In addition, detainment under the Mental Health Act 2007 is increasingly being associated with individuals experiencing trauma (Tarrier et al. 2007). This could relate to treatment being given without consent, as well as frightening hallucinations, all leading to PTSD symptoms (Berry et al. 2013; Swan et al. 2017).

Paramedics and trauma

Given the nature of the work paramedics undertake, it is recognized that PTSD is more common among paramedics when compared to the general population

(Berger et al. 2012; Baqai 2020). This largely results from repeated exposure to chronic and acute experiences, which can lead to a complex aetiology. However, despite this recognition this is largely an under-researched area (Baqai 2020). Berger et al. (2012) reported a 12.6 per cent prevalence in ambulance personnel compared to 1.3–3.5 per cent in the general population. Interestingly, although prevalence is higher than in the general population, paramedics largely do not develop PTSD (Streb et al. 2014). Although it's important to note that not all those exposed to trauma go on to develop PTSD symptoms. Research is ongoing in this important area to understand why some individuals exposed to the same trauma develop PTSD and some don't. The following will explore protective factors as a possible explanation as to why the prevalence of PTSD among paramedics is not significantly higher than the general population.

Protective and risk factors

Protective factors are largely seen as characteristics that lower the risk of negative outcomes or act to reduce risk. Research has identified various risk factors, including, but not limited to, gender, an individual's history of trauma and social support network (Brewin et al. 2000; Streb et al. 2014). Kyron et al. (2021) developed research in this area identifying themes specific to risk and protective factors:

1 cognitive ability
2 personality factors
3 coping propensities
4 peri-traumatic reactions and post-traumatic symptoms
5 workplace factors
6 interpersonal factors
7 events away from work

From these risk and protective factors social support was clearly identified as a protective factor against the development of mental health difficulties (Kyron et al. 2021). Hruska and Barduhn (2021) proposed engagement in recovery activities, as well as identifying meaning as protective factors. The application of such protective factors could therefore act as coping mechanisms (Streb et al. 2014).

Information box 9.11 Sense of coherence

The concept of sense of coherence originates from salutogenesis that operationalized the sense of coherence scale (Antonovsky 1987). Salutogenesis is the source of health, focusing on factors that support health and well-being, as opposed to pathogenesis (Streb et al. 2014). Sense of coherence denotes an individual's ability to use both existing and potential resources to promote well-being and arguably cope with everyday stressors (Streb et al. 2014). Antonovsky (1987) developed a measure of sense of coherence based on an individual's perception of manageability, meaning and comprehensibility.

Research exploring sense of coherence has concluded a negative correlation with PTSD psychopathology (Tagay et al. 2005; Schnyder et al. 2008). In contrast, research also showed a positive correlation with health and life satisfaction (Eriksson and Lindström 2006; Langeland et al. 2007). Therefore, it can be concluded that the greater an individual's sense of coherence the more likely they are to hold the confidence to cope with stressful experiences, including prevention of the development of PTSD (Schnyder et al. 2008; Streb et al. 2014).

Resilience

The field of developmental psychology first applied the term resilience and it has subsequently been widely used to describe an ability to cope with stressors. Resilience is also associated with physical health (Connor et al. 2003). Various definitions of resilience exist, and it is broadly recognized as a multidimensional concept involving thoughts, emotions and behaviours that an individual learns over time (White et al. 2008). Newman (2005) proposed resilience as an individual's ability to adapt to a variety of different experiences that they consider traumatic. Similar to a sense of coherence, Agaibi and Wilson (2005) developed an integrative Person × Situation model that identifies the types of interactions between five clusters of variables: personality, affect regulation, coping, ego defences, and the use of protective factors and resources to support coping.

An individual's resilience can be both learnt and strengthened through engaging with evidence-based interventions such as therapy (Connor et al. 2003). It is important to note that therapy should not be a requirement, and indeed is not necessary for all individuals exposed to repeated trauma. However, service providers do need to provide access to such services if it is required by employees. Resilience can be delivered in other forms, such as through workshops, with a focus on improving coping mechanisms specific to work-related stress (Streb et al. 2014). In addition, this could be integrated into the curriculum.

Conclusion

This chapter has explored some of the key concepts surrounding trauma-informed care from the perspective of the individual and from an organizational context. The causes and consequences of PTSD have been explored, as well as evidence-based interventions. Decision-making specific to pre-hospital care has also been discussed across the life course.

References

Agaibi, C.E. and Wilson, J.P. (2005) Trauma, PTSD and resilience: A review of the literature, *Trauma, Violence and Abuse*, 6(3): 195–216.

Ahmadi, N., Hajsadeghi, F., Mirshkarlo, H.B., Budoff, M., Yehuda, R. and Ebrahimi, R. (2011) Post-traumatic stress disorder, coronary atherosclerosis, and mortality, *American Journal of Cardiology*, 108(1): 29–33.

Alisic, E., Jongmans, M.J., Van Wesel, F. and Kleber, R.J. (2011) Building child trauma theory from longitudinal studies: A meta-analysis, *Clinical Psychology Review*, 31(5): 736–47.

Alisic, E., Tyler, M.P., Giummarra, M.J. et al. (2017) Trauma-informed care for children in the ambulance: International survey among pre-hospital providers, *European Journal of Psychotraumatology*, 8(1): 1273587–8.

American Psychiatric Association (APA) (1980) *Diagnostic and Statistical Manual of Mental Disorders*, 3rd edn. Washington, DC: American Psychiatric Association.

Anacker, C., O'Donnell, K.J. and Meaney, M.J. (2014) Early life adversity and the epigenetic programming of hypothalamic-pituitary-adrenal function, *Dialogues in Clinical Neuroscience*, 16(3): 321–33.

Antonovsky, A. (1987) *Unraveling the Mystery of Health*. San Francisco, CA: Jossey-Bass.

Avraham, N., Goldblatt, H. and Yafe, E. (2014) Paramedics' experiences and coping strategies when encountering critical incidents, *Qualitative Health Research*, 24(2): 194–208.

Baqai, K. (2020) PTSD in paramedics: History, conceptual issues and psychometric measures, *Journal of Paramedic Practice: The Clinical Monthly for Emergency Care Professionals*, 12(12): 495–502.

Benedek, D.M. and Ursano, R.J. (2009) Posttraumatic stress disorder: From phenomenology to clinical practice, *FOCUS: The Journal of Lifelong Learning in Psychiatry*, 7(2): 160–75.

Berger, W., Coutinho, E.S., Figueira, I. et al. (2012) Rescuers at risk: A systematic review and meta-regression analysis of the worldwide current prevalence and correlates of PTSD in rescue workers, *Social Psychiatry and Psychiatric Epidemiology*, 47(6): 1001–11. doi: 10.1007/s00127-011-0408-2.

Berry, K., Ford, S., Jellicoe-Jones, L. and Haddock, G. (2013) PTSD symptoms associated with the experiences of psychosis and hospitalization: A review of the literature, *Clinical Psychology Review*, 33(4): 526–38.

Bienvenu, O.J., Friedman, L.A., Colantuoni, E. et al. (2018) Psychiatric symptoms after acute respiratory distress syndrome: A 5-year longitudinal study, *Intensive Care Medicine*, 44(1): 38–47.

Bienvenu, O.J., Gellar, J., Althouse, B.M. et al. (2013) Post-traumatic stress disorder symptoms after acute lung injury: A 2-year prospective longitudinal study, *Psychological Medicine*, 43(12): 2657–71.

Bisson, J.I. (2007) Post-traumatic stress disorder, *British Medical Journal*, 334(7597): 789–93.

Brewin, C.R., Andrews, B. and Valentine, J.D. (2000) Meta-analysis of risk factors for posttraumatic stress disorder in trauma-exposed adults, *Journal of Consulting and Clinical Psychology*, 68(5): 748–66.

Brymer, M., Layne, C., Jacobs, A. et al. (2006) *Psychological First Aid Field Operations Guide*, 2nd edn. USA: National Child Traumatic Stress Network, National Center for PTSD. Available at: https://www.nctsn.org/resources/psychological-first-aid-pfa-field-operations-guide-2nd-edition (accessed 7 April 2021).

Center for Substance Abuse Treatment (2014) *Trauma-Informed Care in Behavioral Health Services*. Treatment Improvement Protocol Series, No. 57. Rockville, MD: Substance Abuse and Mental Health Services Administration (US) Available at: https://www.ncbi.nlm.nih.gov/books/NBK207201/ (accessed 8 August 2021).

Connor, K.M., Davidson, J.R.T. and Lee, L.-C. (2003) Spirituality, resilience, and anger in survivors of violent trauma: A community survey, *Journal of Traumatic Stress*, 16(5): 487–94.

Cottrell, E.K., O'Brien, K., Curry, M. et al. (2014) Understanding safety in prehospital emergency medical services for children, *Prehospital Emergency Care*, 18(3): 350–8.

Danese, A. and McEwen, B.S. (2012) Adverse childhood experiences, allostasis, allostatic load, and age-related disease, *Physiology and Behaviour*, 106(1): 29–39.

Danese, A., Moffitt, T.E., Harrington, H. et al. (2009) Adverse childhood experiences and adult risk factors for age-related disease: Depression, inflammation, and clustering of metabolic risk markers, *Archives of Paediatrics and Adolescent Medicine*, 163(12): 1135–43.

Davydow, D.S., Gifford, J.M., Desai, S.V., Needham, D.M. and Bienvenu, O.J. (2008) Post-traumatic stress disorder in general intensive care unit survivors: A systematic review, *General Hospital Psychiatry*, 30(5): 421–34.

De Luca, G., Suryapranata, H., Ottervanger, J.P. and Antman, E.M. (2004) Time delay to treatment and mortality in primary angioplasty for acute myocardial infarction: Every minute of delay counts, *Circulation*, 109(10): 1223–5.

Devlin, J.W., Skrobik, Y., Gélinas, C. et al. (2018) Clinical practice guidelines for the prevention and management of pain, agitation/sedation, delirium, immobility, and sleep disruption in adult patients in the ICU, *Critical Care Medicine*, 46(9): e825–73.

Einvik, G., Dammen, T., Ghanima, W., Heir, T. and Stavem, K. (2021) Prevalence and risk factors for post-traumatic stress in hospitalized and non-hospitalized COVID-19 patients, *International Journal of Environmental Research and Public Health*, 18(4): 2079.

Eriksson, M. and Lindström, B. (2006) Antonovsky's sense of coherence scale and the relation with health: A systematic review, *Journal of Epidemiology and Community Health*, 60(5): 376–81. doi: 10.1136/jech.2005.041616.

Fear, N.T., Bridges, S., Hatch, S., Hawkins, V. and Wessely, S. (2016) Posttraumatic stress disorder, in S. McManus, P. Bebbington, R. Jenkins and T. Brugha (eds) *Mental Health and Wellbeing in England: Adult Psychiatric Morbidity Survey*. NHS Digital. Available at: https://files.digital.nhs.uk/pdf/0/8/adult_psychiatric_study_ch4_web.pdf (accessed 8 August 2021).

Filson, B. (2011) 'Is anyone really listening?', *National Council Magazine*, Special Issue: *Breaking the Silence: Trauma-Informed Behavioral Healthcare*, Nos 2/15: 15.

Greene, T., Neria, Y. and Gross, R. (2016) Prevalence, detection and correlates of PTSD in the primary care setting: A systematic review, *Journal of Clinical Psychology in Medical Settings*, 23(2): 160–80.

Gunnarsson, B.-M. and Stomberg, M.W. (2009) Factors influencing decision making among ambulance nurses in emergency care situations, *International Emergency Nursing*, 17(2): 83–9.

Harris, M. and Fallot, R. (2001) *Using Trauma Theory to Design Service Systems: New Directions for Mental Health Services*. San Francisco, CA: Jossey-Bass.

Herman, A.N. and Whitaker, R.C. (2020) Reconciling mixed messages from mixed methods: A randomized trial of a professional development course to increase trauma-informed care, *Child Abuse & Neglect*, 101: 104349.

Hosey, M.M., Leoutsakos, J.S., Li, X. et al. (2019) Screening for posttraumatic stress disorder in ARDS survivors: Validation of the Impact of Event Scale-6 (IES-6), *Critical Care*, 23(1): 276.

Hruska, B. and Barduhn, M.S. (2021) Dynamic psychosocial risk and protective factors associated with mental health in Emergency Medical Service (EMS) personnel, *Journal of Affective Disorders*, 282: 9–17.

Huang, M., Parker, A.M., Bienvenu, O.J. et al. (2016) Psychiatric symptoms in acute respiratory distress syndrome survivors: A one-year national multi-center study, *Critical Care Medicine*, 44(5): 954–65.

Isobel, S. and Edwards, C. (2017) Using trauma informed care as a nursing model of care in an acute inpatient mental health unit: A practice development process, *International Journal of Mental Health Nursing*, 26(1): 88–94.

Jackson, J.C., Jutte, J.E., Hunter, C.H. et al. (2016) Posttraumatic stress disorder (PTSD) after critical illness: A conceptual review of distinct clinical issues and their implications, *Rehabilitation Psychology*, 61(2): 132–40.

Kassam-Adams, N., Marsac, M.L., Hildenbrand, A. and Winston, F. (2013) Posttraumatic stress following pediatric injury: Update on diagnosis, risk factors, and intervention, *JAMA Pediatrics*, 167(12): 1158–65.

Koenen, K.C., Sumner, J.A., Gilsanz, P. et al. (2017) Post-traumatic stress disorder and cardiometabolic disease: Improving causal inference to inform practice, *Psychological Medicine*, 47(2): 209–25.

Kubzansky, L.D., Koenen, K.C., Spiro, A. III, Vokonas, P.S. and Sparrow, D. (2007) Prospective study of posttraumatic stress disorder symptoms and coronary heart disease in the Normative Aging Study, *Archives of General Psychiatry*, 64(1): 109–16.

Kyron, M.J., Rees, C.S., Lawrence, D., Carleton, R.N. and McEvoy, P.M. (2021) Prospective risk and protective factors for psychopathology and wellbeing in civilian emergency services personnel: A systematic review, *Journal of Affective Disorders*, 281: 517–32.

Langeland, E., Wahl, A.K., Kristoffersen, K., Nortvedt, M.W. and Hanestad, B.R. (2007) Sense of coherence predicts change in life satisfaction among home-living residents in the community with mental health problems: A 1-year follow-up study, *Quality of Life Research*, 16(6): 939–46. doi: 10.1007/s11136-007-9199-z.

Lasiuk G.C. and Hegadoren K.M. (2006) Posttraumatic stress disorder part I: Historical development of the concept, *Perspectives in Psychiatric Care*, 42(1): 13–20.

Lehavot, K., Goldberg, S.B., Chen, J.A. et al. (2018) Do trauma type, stressful life events, and social support explain women veterans' high prevalence of PTSD?, *Social Psychiatry and Psychiatric Epidemiology*, 53(9): 943–53.

Lohr, J.B., Palmer, B.W., Eidt, C.A. et al. (2015) Is post-traumatic stress disorder associated with premature senescence? A review of the literature, *American Journal of Geriatric Psychiatry*, 23(7): 709–25.

Lomanowska, A.M., Boivin, M., Hertzman, C. and Fleming A.S. (2017) Parenting begets parenting: A neurobiological perspective on early adversity and the transmission of parenting styles across generations, *Neuroscience*, 342: 120–39.

Lommen, M.J.J. and Restifo, K. (2009) Trauma and posttraumatic stress disorder (PTSD) in patients with schizophrenia or schizoaffective disorder, *Community Mental Health Journal*, 45(6): 485–96.

Magruder, K.M., Kassam-Adams, N., Thoresen, S. and Olff, M. (2016) Prevention and public health approaches to trauma and traumatic stress: A rationale and a call to action, *European Journal of Psychotraumatology*, 7(1): 29715.

Maniglio, R. (2009) Severe mental illness and criminal victimization: A systematic review, *Acta Psychiatrica Scandinavica*, 119(3): 180–91.

Marsac, M.L., Kassam-Adams, N., Delahanty, D.L., Widaman, K.F. and Barakat, L.P. (2014) Posttraumatic stress following acute medical trauma in children: A proposed model of bio-psycho-social processes during the peri-trauma period, *Clinical Child and Family Psychology Review*, 17(4): 399–411.

Mersky, J.P., Topitzes, J. and Reynolds, A.J. (2013) Impacts of adverse childhood experiences on health, mental health, and substance use in early adulthood: A cohort study of an urban, minority sample in the US, *Child Abuse & Neglect*, 37(11): 917–25.

Newman, J.D., Muntner, P., Shimbo, D., Davidson, K.W., Shaffer, J.A. and Edmondson, D. (2011) Post-traumatic stress disorder (PTSD) symptoms predict delay to hospital in patients with acute coronary syndrome, *PloS one*, 6(11): e27640.

Newman, R. (2005) APA's resilience initiative, *Professional Psychology: Research and Practice*, 36(3): 227–9.

National Institute for Health and Care Excellence (NICE) (2018) *Post-Traumatic Stress Disorder*. NICE guideline NG116. London: NICE.

Nordén, C., Hult, K. and Engström, Å. (2014) Ambulance nurses' experiences of nursing critically ill and injured children: A difficult aspect of ambulance nursing care, *International Emergency Nursing*, 22(2): 75–80.

Öberg, M., Vicente, V. and Wahlberg, A.C. (2015) The Emergency Medical Service personnel's perception of the transportation of young children, *International Emergency Nursing*, 23: 133–7.

Oral, R., Coohey, C., Zarei, K. et al. (2020) Nationwide efforts for trauma-informed care implementation and workforce development in healthcare and related fields: A systematic review, *Turkish Journal of Paediatrics*, 62(6): 906–20.

Parker, A.M., Sricharoenchai, T., Raparla, S., Schneck, K.W., Bienvenu, O.J. and Needham, D.M. (2015) Posttraumatic stress disorder in critical illness survivors: A metanalysis, *Critical Care Medicine*, 43(5): 1121–9.

Read, J., Hammersley, P. and Rudegeair, T. (2007) Why, when and how to ask about childhood abuse, *Advances in Psychiatric Treatment*, 13(2): 101–10.

Roberts, A.L., Agnew-Blais, J.C., Spiegelman, D. et al. (2015) Posttraumatic stress disorder and incidence of type 2 diabetes mellitus in a sample of women: A 22-year longitudinal study, *JAMA Psychiatry*, 72(3): 203–10.

Salasin S. (2011) Sine qua non for public health, *National Council Magazine*, 18.

Schnyder, U., Wittmann, L., Friedrich-Perez, J., Hepp, U. and Moergeli, H. (2008) Posttraumatic stress disorder following accidental injury: Rule or exception in Switzerland?, *Psychotherapy and Psychosomatics*, 77(2): 111–18. doi: 10.1159/000112888.

Shapiro, F. (2001) *Eye Movement Desensitization and Reprocessing: Basic Principles, Protocols, and Procedures*. New York: Guilford Press.

Shemesh, E., Yehuda, R., Milo, O. et al. (2004) Posttraumatic stress, nonadherence, and adverse outcome in survivors of a myocardial infarction, *Psychosomatic Medicine*, 66(4): 521–6.

Shonkoff, J.P., Garner, A.S., Siegel, B.S. et al. (2012) The lifelong effects of early childhood adversity and toxic stress, *Paediatrics*, 129(1): e232–46.

Smolderen, K.G., Spertus, J.A., Nallamothu, B.K. et al. (2010) Health Care Insurance, Financial Concerns in Accessing Care, and Delays to Hospital Presentation in Acute Myocardial Infarction, *JAMA*, 303(14): 1392–400.

Streb, M., Häller, P. and Michael, T. (2014) PTSD in paramedics: Resilience and sense of coherence, *Behavioural and Cognitive Psychotherapy*, 42(4): 452–63.

Stuber, M.L., Schneider, S., Kassam-Adams, N., Kazak, A. E. and Saxe, G. (2006) The medical traumatic stress toolkit, *CNS Spectrums*, 11(2): 137–42.

Sun, J., Patel, F., Rose-Jacobs, R., Frank, D.A., Black, M.M. and Chilton, M. (2017) Mothers' adverse childhood experiences and their young children's development, *American Journal of Preventive Medicine*, 53(6): 882–91.

Swan, S., Keen, N., Reynolds, N. and Onwumere, J. (2017) Psychological interventions for post-traumatic stress symptoms in psychosis: A systematic review of outcomes, *Frontiers in Psychology*, 8: 341.

Sweeney, A., Clement, S., Filson, B. and Kennedy, A. (2016) Trauma-informed mental healthcare in the UK: What is it and how can we further its development?, *Mental Health Review Journal*, 21(3): 174–92.

Tagay, S., Herpertz, S., Langkafel, M. and Senf, W. (2005) Posttraumatic stress disorder in a psychosomatic outpatient clinic: Gender effects, psychosocial functioning, sense of coherence, and service utilization, *Journal of Psychosomatic Research*, 58: 439–46. doi: 10.1016/j.jpsychores. 2004.09.007.

Tarrier, N., Khan, S., Cater, J. and Picken, A. (2007) The subjective consequences of suffering a first episode psychosis: Trauma and suicide behavior, *Social Psychiatry and Psychiatric Epidemiology*, 42(1): 29–35.

Ting, H.H., Bradley, E.H., Wang, Y. et al. (2008) Factors associated with longer time from symptom onset to hospital presentation for patients with ST-elevation myocardial infarction, *Archives of Internal Medicine*, 168(9): 959–68.

Ting, H.H., Chen, A.Y., Roe, M.T. et al. (2010) Delay from symptom onset to hospital presentation for patients with non-ST-segment elevation myocardial infarction, *Archives of Internal Medicine*, 170(20): 1834–41.

Trickey, D., Siddaway, A.P., Meiser-Stedman, R., Serpell, L. and Field, A.P. (2012) A meta-analysis of risk factors for post-traumatic stress disorder in children and adolescents, *Clinical Psychology Review*, 32(2): 122–38.

Vaccarino, V., Goldberg, J., Magruder, K.M. et al. (2014) Posttraumatic stress disorder and incidence of type-2 diabetes: A prospective twin study, *Journal of Psychiatric Research*, 56: 158–64.

Walczewska, J., Rutkowski, K., Wizner, B., Cwynar, M. and Grodzicki, T. (2010) Stiffness of large arteries and cardiovascular risk in patients with post-traumatic stress disorder, *European Heart Journal*, 32(6): 730–6.

White, B., Driver, S. and Warren, A. (2008) Considering resilience in the rehabilitation of people with traumatic disabilities, *Rehabilitation Psychology*, 53(1): 9–17.

Williamson, V. and Greenberg, N. (2019) Post-traumatic stress disorder: Diagnosis and management, *Trends in Urology & Men's Health*, 10(4): 14–16.

Wilson, A. and Beresford, P. (2002) Madness, distress and postmodernity: Putting the record straight, in M. Corker and T. Shakespeare (eds) *Disability/Postmodernity: Embodying Disability Theory*. New York: Continuum, pp. 143–58.

World Health Organization (2018) *International Classification of Diseases for Mortality and Morbidity Statistics* (11th revision) [online]. Available at: https://icd.who.int/browse11/l-m/en (accessed 8 April 2021).

Further reading

Magruder, K.M., Kassam-Adams, N., Thoresen, S. and Olff, M. (2016) Prevention and public health approaches to trauma and traumatic stress: A rationale and a call to action, *European Journal of Psychotraumatology*, 7(1): 29715.

Read, J., Hammersley, P. and Rudegeair, T. (2007) Why, when and how to ask about childhood abuse, *Advances in Psychiatric Treatment*, 13(2): 101–10.

10 Conclusion

Jo Augustus, Yuet Wah Patrick and Paula Gardner

Paramedic science: the current position

As a profession, paramedic science is an essential part of medicine, and has seen a recent diversification of career paths, for example within primary care. The authors recognize that paramedics are increasingly encountering complex mental health difficulties in practice and needing to provide the most appropriate care pathway. In order to do this, they require an effective understanding of mental health and evidence-based practice in the context of emergency medicine, which the authors have sought to address in this book. Some of the underpinning themes in the book have included the bio-psycho-social model applied across the life course, person-centred practice, as well as evidence-based medicine. These themes have provided a framework to explore:

- Legislation principles and practices within the wider context of multidisciplinary working
- The key characteristics of a variety of different mental health difficulties, integrated into the assessment processes
- Complex mental health needs, addressed through the lens of the bio-psycho-social model
- An understanding of evidence-based practice and the provision of person-centred care in the context of referral pathways
- Trauma-informed care in organizational contexts

The education and training of paramedics has increasingly diversified beyond emergency medicine. Consequently the curriculum has expanded to include subjects aligned to primary and secondary care, in addition to broader public health themes. Arguably this has sought to address the needs of paramedics practising in contemporary healthcare (O'Meara et al. 2017). Paramedic practitioner roles have seen a development in career paths available, responding to changing population needs – for example an increasingly aging population, in addition to the prevalence of chronic conditions (Keady et al. 2013). This diversification of education and training has seen a move towards a model of holistic care provision, while being both flexible and responsive to patient needs (O'Meara et al. 2017). To the future, an increase in the use of interprofessional learning is expected to support collaboration and clinical reasoning as well as the development of technical skills (Shields and Flin 2013; Bennett et al. 2021). This may include clinical simulation to provide meaningful learning opportunities from learning environments, transferable into practice (Yule et al. 2018; Murray et al. 2019).

Paramedic science: the future

As the profession of paramedic science continues to evolve, paramedics remain the first point of contact in the provision of evidence-based practice. This includes working autonomously in the assessment and treatment of individuals experiencing a variety of difficulties including mental health (Shields and Flin 2013). This is especially pertinent to the provision of care in a post-COVID-19 world. This book has sought to provide paramedics with essential information specific to the theory and practice surrounding mental health (Carley et al. 2020).

References

Bennett, R., Mehmed, N. and Williams, B. (2021) Non-technical skills in paramedicine: A scoping review, *Nursing and Health Sciences*, 23(1): 40–52.

Carley, S., Horner, D., Body, R. and Mackway-Jones, K. (2020) Evidence-based medicine and COVID-19: What to believe and when to change, *Emergency Medicine Journal*, 37(9): 572–5.

Keady, J., Jones, L., Ward, R. et al. (2013) Introducing the bio-psycho-social-physical model of dementia through a collective case study design, *Journal of Clinical Nursing*, 22(19–20): 2768–77.

Murray, B., Judge, D., Morris, T. and Opsahl, A. (2019) Interprofessional education: A disaster response simulation activity for military medics, nursing, & paramedic science students, *Nurse Education in Practice*, 39: 67–72.

O'Meara, P.F., Furness, S. and Gleeson, R. (2017) Educating paramedics for the future: A holistic approach, *Journal of Health and Human Services Administration*, 40(2): 219–51.

Shields, A. and Flin, R. (2013) Paramedics' non-technical skills: A literature review, *Emergency Medicine Journal*, 30(5): 350–4.

Yule, S., Gupta, A., Gazarian, D. et al. (2018) Construct and criterion validity testing of the non-technical skills for surgeons (NOTSS) behaviour assessment tool using videos of simulated operations, *British Journal of Surgery*, 105(6): 719–27.

Glossary

Abnormal psychology
A branch of psychology that studies unusual patterns of behaviour, thoughts and emotions, that may be conceptualized as a mental health diagnosis.

Aetiology
The causes or origin of disease, including factors that predispose an individual towards a certain disease or disorder.

Assessment
The process of gathering information to evaluate an individual's behaviour, capabilities and other characteristics, for the purpose of making a diagnosis or treatment recommendation.

Bio-psycho-social model
The bio-psycho-social model encompasses multidimensional components relevant to the individual's biological, psychological and social factors, and the interconnection between these.

Common mental health problems
Mild to moderate presentation of anxiety and depression-related diagnoses that are considered to have a moderate impact on day-to-day functioning. This includes depression and anxiety disorders such as generalized anxiety disorder, panic disorder, obsessive-compulsive disorder and post-traumatic stress disorder.

Contraindicator
A clinical rationale to not administer a certain medical treatment due to the harm that it would cause the patient.

Diagnostic criteria
Contain descriptions, symptoms and other criteria for diagnosing mental disorders.

Evidence-based practice
The integration of best available research evidence that combines clinical expertise and patient values.

Maladaptive coping strategies
Unhelpful coping strategies used by individuals to cope with difficult experiences, providing short-term relief. Examples include dissociation, avoidance and escape self-medication.

Mental health
A state of well-being in which an individual understands their own abilities, can cope with everyday life stress, can work productively and can contribute to their community.

Person-centred care
The provision of care coordinated in collaboration with and tailored to an individual's needs.

Post-traumatic stress disorder
Following exposure to an extremely threatening or horrific event or series of events, individuals may re-experience the event through vivid intrusive memories, flashbacks or nightmares, and may experience avoidance of association and/or a sense of heightened current threat.

Pre-hospital care
The care services a patient receives from emergency services prior to hospital admission, if this is required. This may include assessment, stabilization and transportation to an appropriate service.

Primary care
Primary care services provide the first point of contact to healthcare, including the NHS. Primary care includes general practice, community pharmacy, dental and optometry services.

Resilience
The capacity an individual has to adapt to and/or recover from adversity, such as loss and change, trauma or significant stress.

Risk assessment
The process of evaluating risk of harm to self or others, which includes consideration of medical, psychological and social factors specific to the individual.

Secondary care
Secondary care encompasses specialist service providers, and includes both hospital and community care. It may be planned or involve urgent and emergency care.

Severe and enduring mental health problems
Individuals experiencing chronic and long-term symptoms that significantly impair their day-to-day functioning. This includes, but is not limited to, bipolar disorder, schizophrenia, self-harm, eating disorders and personality disorder.

Trauma
The psychological response to an extremely threatening or horrific event or series of events.

Trauma-informed care
A framework for service delivery that is equipped with the knowledge, skills and understanding of how trauma impacts on an individual or individuals.

Index

Page numbers with 't' are tables; with 'b' are boxes; with 'g' are glossary terms.